FUNCTIONAL ASSESSMENT
IN MASSAGE THERAPY
Third Edition

A guide to orthopedic assessment of pain and injury conditions for the massage practioner.

Whitney W. Lowe, LMT

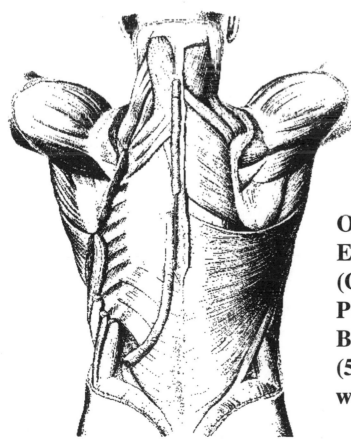

Published by:

**Orthopedic Massage
Education & Research Institute
(OMERI)
PO Box 1468
Bend, OR 97709
(541) 317-9855
www.omeri.com**

For additional copies of the book
and information about OMERI
contact:

Orthopedic Massage Education &
Research Institute (OMERI)
PO Box 1468
Bend, OR 97709
tel. (541) 317-9855
fax (541) 317-9856
www.omeri.com
wlowe@omeri.com

ISBN 0-9661196-0-6

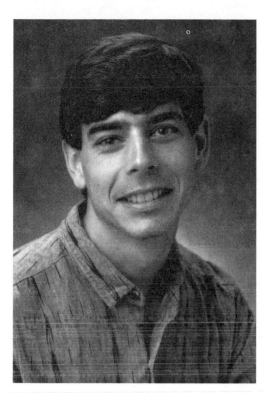

About the Author

Whitney Lowe is one of the most dynamic educators in the massage therapy field. He researches and writes articles on pain and injury assessment techniques in national journals and in his bi-monthly research newsletter, Orthopedic & Sports Massage Reviews. Lowe co-developed the Clinical Sports Massage Program at the Atlanta School of Massage, a 620 hour program specifically devoted to treating soft-tissue pain and injuries with massage therapy. While in Atlanta he developed a strong academic background including graduate study in psychology, sports medicine and biomechanics. He teaches workshops nationally and internationally on orthopedic massage and assessment skills. Lowe is the owner and director of the Orthopedic Massage Education & Research Institute, headquartered in Bend, Oregon.

This publication is designed to be an educational resource and should not be considered as a substitute for proper training in the methods contained herein. In using any techniques presented in this book, the practitioner is encouraged to use sound clinical judgement and a healthy dose of common sense. As a health care practitioner you will always encounter conditions that will fall outside your area of expertise. It is your responsibility to make well educated decisions about the limits of your training and ability to help each individual.

Dedication

To my family:
An inspirational group of artists and scholars
who have all taught me so much.

Acknowledgements

This book was made possible by the contributions of many individuals. I have been fortunate to have many great teachers, friends, and colleagues who have been an integral part of the production. I would like to offer a special thanks to Elise Wolf for her crucial feedback and wonderful companionship and to Benny Vaughn who has been an invaluable mentor and friend. Thanks to Rick Garbowski for help with the illustrations, proofreading, and brainstorming, Johnny Reed for assistance in proofreading, Louann Nannini, Doug Beasley, and Darrah Levick for assistance with the illustrations, the staff of the Emory Clinic Sports Medicine Center, and the faculty and staff of the Atlanta School of Massage. Thanks very much to Grace Eckert of Educational Graphics for the time and effort involved in creating some of the illustrations that were used in the book. These images are available as a separate slide program. Information about the slide program can be obtained from Educational Graphics at: PO Box 10793, Reno, NV 89510. Thanks to the staff of the Corvallis, Oregon Kinko's computer lab for their help in the technical preparation of the book. I would also like to thank all the many massage practitioners, educators, and students who I have met across the country whose valuable input and feedback helped form the ideas that molded the book.

Foreword

As a practicing Licensed Massage Therapist since 1975 I have always been concerned about evaluating and assessing muscle, tendon, and ligament complaints that I saw with my clients. My massage therapy training in 1974 was void of functional assessment skills, as was every other massage school curriculum in the United States. Consequently, I returned to college to become a Certified Athletic Trainer. Orthopedic assessment is a major component of the skills that Certified Athletic Trainers are required to master, primarily to work with injured athletes.

While working as a Massage Therapist and Athletic Trainer it became increasingly apparent to me that massage therapists should have at their disposal solid training in fundamental orthopedic assessment skills. It is, in my view, one of the key factors to moving massage therapy into the health care delivery system as an equal partner to traditional Western therapies in treating soft-tissue problems and concerns, rather than as just an adjunctive modality.

For over a decade now, I have taught and promoted orthopedic functional assessment skills to massage therapists -- in workshops, seminars, and massage school trainings across the United States. All along I had to resort to a collection of injury assessment and physical examination textbooks that were written for medical doctors, athletic trainers, and physical therapists. There were no textbooks or manuals available that presented orthopedic assessment with massage therapy in mind. That has now changed because of Whitney Lowe, who first came to my attention as a participant in one of my weekend workshop programs in Atlanta, Georgia.

Whitney Lowe has authored, in my opinion, the best manual of orthopedic assessment designed specifically for massage therapy. This manual takes the mystery out of orthopedic assessment by providing descriptions and characteristics of conditions likely to be encountered by massage therapists. The reader is then provided with suggestions for treatment and care utilizing massage therapy.

Functional Assessment in Massage Therapy is a terrific single source working manual for any massage therapist working with people who have muscle, tendon, and ligament complaints. It is written by a massage therapist for massage therapists and can provide an important step in improving the level of massage care that a practitioner can provide. By knowing what type of musculoskeletal condition you have encountered, your ability to administer the appropriate massage therapy protocol for the best results is greatly enhanced. This manual is an investment in achieving success with your massage therapy clients.

Benny F. Vaughn, LMT, ATC, CSCS
Atlanta, Georgia

Preface to the 3rd edition

During the course of teaching massage therapy students in many different educational environments, it became evident to me that additional training resources for working with soft-tissue injuries were badly needed. This book has been a constantly evolving educational resource designed to fit the many needs of massage practitioners working with soft-tissue injuries. In this edition there are numerous illustrations to help describe the injury conditions and make the information more understandable for those who are visual learners. The format and content are mostly consistent with the second edition, with the exception of a few minor changes and corrections.

It is my feeling that the learning of assessment skills is an on-going practice. This reference book is designed to be one step along the way to learning assessment. There is no substitute for actual hands-on learning and the benefit of seeing some of these situations in "real life". I encourage the reader to keep an open mind when assessing soft-tissue problems. Unfortunately there is no reliable "recipe" book of exactly how to do it. Much of your skill in assessment and treatment will rely on practice, common sense, and the skills that are developed with experience.

Whitney W. Lowe, L.M.T.
Bend, Oregon
October, 1997

Contents

Section One

Theoretical Principles of Assessment

Section Two
Conditions and Assessment
by Anatomical Region

Section 1
Theoretical Principles
of Assessment

CHAPTER 1

INTRODUCTION TO FUNCTIONAL ASSESSMENT

The use of therapeutic massage to treat soft-tissue pain conditions is rapidly gaining acceptance across many divergent regions of the health care landscape. Although the majority of health care practitioners performing therapeutic massage are known as massage therapists, other professionals such as nurses, chiropractors, physical therapists, osteopathic physicians, or athletic trainers may also use many of the same treatment methods. Throughout this book the term *massage therapy* will be used to refer to the use of massage to treat various pathological conditions of the soft-tissues. The term massage therapist will be used as a general reference to the practitioner of massage regardless of his or her specialty.

Education and training in the use of massage therapy varies greatly across the country. Some allied health care specialties such as physical therapy or athletic training incorporate rudimentary massage principles into their curriculum. However, the development of massage technique has advanced so far as to make most of these courses just a superficial introduction. The unfortunate outcome of this is that many allied health care professionals develop a limited view of what can be accomplished with the use of massage therapy because their view of massage is based primarily on a limited exposure.

Massage therapists generally have less academic "medically oriented" training than many of these other specialists. They have a great deal of instruction in numerous methods of massage which reduce pain and help alleviate soft-tissue dysfunction. The high level of success which many massage therapists have achieved with different soft-tissue pain conditions has led to a greater demand for this therapeutic service by the general public. Unfortunately, because of the lack of adequate academic training, many massage therapists are unable to explain exactly why they get the results they get. This will often lead to exaggerated claims about the effectiveness of massage and an inaccurate picture of how best to apply these valuable treatment methods.

By not understanding the nature of various injuries and the physiological effects of certain methods of massage, all practitioners of massage therapy may limit their effectiveness. If massage is inappropriately used, a well-meaning practitioner may not only be ineffective, he/she may in fact cause harm. An important part of the Hippocratic oath taken by medical practitioners since the time of the ancient Greeks is: *above all, do no harm.* Massage practitioners should remember this and always keep the client's best interest in mind.

Keeping the client's health and well-being foremost in mind is important since massage therapists and some other practitioners of massage are direct access providers. This means that a person can walk in off the street to a massage therapist and request care for a particular condition. The massage therapist can then offer treatment to that person without a referral or prescription from any other health provider. Many allied health care providers do not have this ability. While direct access is a wonderful opportunity for the client and massage practitioner alike, there is an increased responsibility that comes with it. Massage practitioners who enjoy direct access must have some form of assessment skills in order to determine if each client's condition is something that could be helped by massage.

Massage practitioners, while often taught many different methods for treating soft-tissue dysfunction, rarely learn the skills necessary to determine what condition(s) is/are present. One of the best ways to determine the nature of various conditions and the appropriate choice of treatment methods is through the use of assessment skills. The assessment approach presented in this book will focus on orthopedic disorders. The term orthopedic refers to those problems which are directly related to the locomotor system of the body. The responsibility of the locomotor system is to create or limit movement. Therefore orthopedic problems are those that involve the creation or limitation of movement. Many people don't realize that the limitation (deceleration) of motion is just as important as the creation (acceleration) of motion. In fact, it is often the deceleration of movement that is primarily responsible for causing soft-tissue injury. This will become clear later on as we discuss eccentric muscle contractions and the mechanical forces that biological tissues are subjected to.

There are some systems of assessment which promote the use of various muscle testing procedures to evaluate the function of organ systems or organic/chemical balances in the body. Some practitioners may use this "muscle testing" to evaluate all types of other problems in the body such as a person's allergic reactions to specific foods. Those methods are considered outside the scope of this book. In this text, we will focus attention on those tissues involved in creating and limiting movement and how they can be evaluated and treated by massage therapy.

Assessment skills have historically not been an important part of massage education for several reasons. The current interest in massage therapy in this country developed out of the human potential movement of the 1960's and 70's. At first, education in this field focused on the use of massage as another means of becoming more aware of the physical body. It was not used very often to treat pathological conditions other than general stress and tension. As the profession has grown, massage practitioners have greatly improved their skills and knowledge, and applied these abilities to the treatment of various soft-tissue disorders. However, adequate educational resources and training methods for assessment skills have not yet become a part of most education programs.

The growing profession of massage therapy has emerged alongside the surge of interest in alternative systems of health care. The strength of many of these alternative systems are open-minded paradigms of the healing potential of the human body. Many of the practitioners in the alternative or holistic health community have gravitated there because of their dissatisfaction with the traditional "mainstream" medical establishment. The ground-breaking article on unconventional medicine in the U.S. in the January 1993 issue of *The New England Journal of Medicine* is evidence of a major shift in awareness and use of these various alternative and complimentary therapies. However, many of the practitioners of these alternative systems have developed a corresponding negative attitude and mind-set about anything that seems too "medical" or "mainstream health care". One should be cautious about "throwing the baby out with the bath water". The systematic procedures for testing function of the locomotor soft-tissues presented in this book come directly from established "mainstream medi-cal" models. They are, however, highly useful and completely adaptable to the holistic models under which most massage therapists operate.

One of the reasons orthopedic assessment skills are not adequately taught is because many massage practitioners misunderstand the concept of assessment. Massage therapists, for example, are continually reminded that they are not to diagnose any condition. While that is absolutely correct, that does not mean they should not assess each individual situation. If a client comes to a massage practitioner and wishes to be treated for a soft tissue injury, that practitioner has a responsibility to determine if the condition is appropriately treated by massage, or if it should be referred to another health care professional. Without some form of assessment skills it becomes very difficult, if not impossible, for the practitioner to make a sound decision about how, or if, this person should be treated. This is one of the most important and basic reasons why assessment skills should be taught in entry level massage training programs.

There is a distinct difference between assessment and diagnosis. A diagnosis is an assigned name or label for an existing condition that is provided by a qualified health care provider such as a physician. Assessment is an on-going process of information gathering that is used to help in making clinical decisions. As a massage practitioner, you will be using assessment skills throughout the duration of your treatment in order to determine if your approach is having a beneficial effect. A physician may use information gathered during assessment to make a diagnosis, but the process of assessment in and of itself is not diagnosis. A massage practitioner will use assessment skills to evaluate the nature of his/her client's complaint and continually insure that the current approach or method of treatment is the most effective for each individual.

> *Functional assessment skills are systematic problem solving methods that will give the massage practitioner a sound basis for making educated decisions about treatment with massage.*

In addition to determining if a condition should be treated by massage, functional assessment skills are very helpful in managing the course of treatment. It often happens that during treatment the practitioner will have to make judgements about whether the current approach is getting the desired results. If the desired results are not being produced, it is obvious that the course of treatment needs to be modified. The initial evaluation can provide a baseline against which progress can be measured. On-going assessment will help the practitioner fully understand the progress of each individual's condition.

Specific methods of measuring progress will become very important as the effectiveness of massage therapy is studied through clinical research. Clinical research is important to understand the experiences that practitioners have with massage. The efficacy of massage therapy as a viable mode of health care will rest strongly on the results of these investigative studies. The ability to have massage therapy covered under various health insurance plans will also depend on the specifically measurable results attained from these studies.

As you learn various skills of assessment, remember that the use of these skills is both an art and a science. There is a specific rationale that follows certain rules and protocols. That is the science. However, there are very few black and white answers, and often it is the intuitive, artistic, and imaginative side of our brain which is more effective at synthesizing feedback from our evaluations and determining how to use that information. That is the art. Functional assessment skills will need to be continually practiced and refined in order for you to get the best use of them.

The Foundations of Soft-Tissue Pathology

One of the primary factors that brings any client in to see a massage practitioner is that they are in pain or discomfort. That pain or discomfort may not necessarily be severe or debilitating, and it may take the form of just tension or mild discomfort. However, it is still the signal of something that is not right in the body and the client's attention will be continually drawn to that area. This, in fact, is one of the distinct advantages that massage practitioners may utilize to their benefit. We offer a form of treatment which in most cases will provide immediate results and feedback (usually through a reduction in pain) on how our treatment has affected the client and their condition.

The pain that we feel in the soft tissues is usually an indicator of some type of pathology or disturbance to normal function in the localized area where the pain is felt. However, there are some important exceptions which will be discussed in the following sections. An effective way to look at soft-tissue dysfunction and pain is by examining what is happening in the tissues. This can be done by dividing the problem into one of two categories - mechanical disruption of tissue and neurological dysfunction. Remember that the nature of categories are inherently limiting and they should not be considered as rigid structures. They are invented by us in order to help us understand complex concepts. Therefore you will often encounter conditions which have characteristics of both of these categories. The purpose of the categories will simply be to give you a way to organize the information that you process during your assessment.

Pain conditions and soft-tissue dysfunction may be of an acute or chronic nature. An acute pain or injury is one that happened all at once. There is a direct link between some event and the immediate onset of pain. An example of an acute injury/pain would be stepping off a curb and twisting your ankle. (This is a common mechanism of an inversion ankle sprain and most likely will cause an injury to the anterior talofibular ligament). The cause of an acute injury is often more easy to identify because the person can usually remember significant details about the event. These details will be crucial for the practitioner when gathering information about an acute injury.

Chronic injuries or pain conditions are often more problematic because it is harder to pinpoint their exact cause. A chronic injury is often called an "overuse condition" or an "overuse syndrome." In a chronic injury, there is a repetitive overstressing of certain anatomical structures that eventually leads to that structure's degeneration. This may happen over a long period of time (several years) or over a relatively short period of time (a day or even an hour). However, the primary characteristic is that there was not just a single movement which caused the injury, but a cumulative effect of many movements which were taxing on the anatomical structures involved. An example is carpal tunnel syndrome. Excessive use of the hand and finger flexor muscles with the wrist in a poor anatomical position leads to compression of the median nerve in the carpal tunnel. With chronic injuries, it is not the effect of a single movement which causes the injury, but the repeated cumulative effect compiled over time.

1. Mechanical Disruption of Tissue

A thorough understanding of the nature of soft-tissue injury and dysfunction of the locomotor tissues will require an awareness of some basic concepts from mechanical physics. Physics has a tendency to be intimidating to many people, but these fundamental concepts of mechanical physics are really quite simple. In fact we interact with these concepts dozens of times every day. The mechanical disruption of soft-tissues comes about because of their exposure to excessive forces. A force may be thought of as either a push or a pull. It is something that will tend to cause a change in motion or shape of an object or body. Most of us have an inherent knowledge of what a force is but we have a hard time putting it into words. Understanding the application of mechanical forces to the body will greatly enhance your ability to determine the nature of various injury conditions.

An examination of how forces interact with the body can help illustrate the nature of these forces in creating soft-tissue injury. The tissues of the human body, just like the metal and concrete in a building, are susceptible to five different types of mechanical forces: compression, tension, torsion, bending, and shear. We will define each of these five types of mechanical force. In determining what causes soft-tissue injuries we will be most interested in compression and tension.

Compression- is when two structures are pressed together. When that force is greater than the structural stability of the materials making up the object (tissue in this case), some type of breakdown of the tissue may occur. An example of a compression injury is a bruise that happens as the result of a direct impact to your muscle tissue. The capillary walls are crushed in the impact and blood leaks out into the cellular spaces creating the discoloration you see and know as ecchymosis or a bruise.

Tension- is the pulling apart of a structure. In this instance there are two opposing forces that are exerting a tensile (pulling) force on a substance (soft-tissue for example). In the body, a tensile stress injury may occur from one force that pulls two ends of a tissue away from each other. An example is a knee ligament injury where a force to the knee causes the two ends of a ligament, which are firmly attached to bony segments, to be pulled away from each other. The tissue will usually stretch to a certain degree before it tears.

Torsion- is a special type of stress that is applied in a rotary or twisting fashion. Torsion may create increased tension or compression as it is applied. Because the soft-tissues are so pliable they are somewhat resistant to torsion stress. Torsion stress affects rigid structures like the bones more than the soft-tissues.

Bending- is actually a combination of compression and tension. One side of a substance or tissue is being compressed while another side is under tension. Bending can be considered the result of applying a force to a region that does not have a stabilizing support. Soft-tissues, again because of their pliability, do not often develop injuries that are the result of bending stress. The bones are much more susceptible to bending stress because they are a rigid structure. An example of bending stress can be illustrated with something called a boot-top fracture that happens to snow skiers. The snow skier wears a rigid boot that comes up above the ankle and fastens tightly to the ski. If the skier falls over forward and the ski stays on the ground, the front side of the tibia will be compressed while the back side of the tibia will be under tensile stress. A bone can only bend up until a certain point before it will break. This is a common mechanism of bone fractures.

Shear- is a force that is best described as a sliding force between two tissues. It is very much like the action between the two blades of a scissors. Soft-tissues are not often injured from shear stress. It takes a good deal of shear to cause trauma to the soft-tissues because of their pliability. However certain regions may be exposed to shear stress that will impact the adjacent or supporting soft-tissues. Spondylolisthesis, is a sliding of one vertebra in relation to the sacrum or another vertebra. This is an example of shear stress.

When a tissue is exposed to one of these forces it will resist the force to a certain degree. Most of the soft-tissues have a certain degree of pliability so their ability to withstand certain forces is often greater. However, if a tissue is subjected to a force that is greater than its ability to absorb that force, the tissue is overloaded and will be damaged. If, for example, a muscle is stretched, it will respond to that stretch by elongating. A certain amount of elongating will be within that muscle's normal ability to lengthen. However, after a certain point, if that muscle is continually stretched, the fibers will not be able to withstand the tensile stress (tension) and the muscle will tear. This is what happens in a muscle strain. It is best to remember that all the soft-tissues have an ability to withstand certain forces, but excessive amounts of force will cause those tissues to be damaged.

Tissues may be subjected to these excessive loads in one of two different ways. They may be suddenly overloaded, which will produce an acute injury, or they may be repeatedly loaded, which will produce a chronic injury. An important factor to remember about chronic injuries is that the load can be very small and still cause an injury. The damage results from a load being applied over and over again. It is the same as if you take a small strip of metal and bend it back and forth in your hands. Bending it one time is not likely to damage it significantly. However, if you keep doing it over and over again, soon it will break.

The various soft tissues will respond to these different mechanical forces in a similar fashion. The body has a complex and well developed system for coping with the mechanical stresses that cause tissue disruption. When an injury occurs that disrupts the continuity of the tissue, the body will immediately try to repair that region of tissue disruption. It does not matter if the disruption happened as the result of an acute or a chronic injury. In either event, the body will develop scar tissue to repair that region. This development of scar tissue is an excellent way of binding together the torn ends of damaged fibers. The drawback to the injury repair process is that often the body produces too much scar tissue or allows it to form in places that actually limit function and may eventually make the condition worse. An example is scar tissue that adheres a healing ligament to the underlying bone. The scar tissue is valuable in binding together the torn ends of the ligament but adhering the ligament to the underlying bone will limit the functional mobility of the joint. The limitation to functional mobility may lead to other mechanical compensations such as muscle shortening and altered joint mechanics.

The primary rationale for the use of massage therapy is to manage the development of scar tissue. It must be remembered that the goal of the massage treatment is not to get rid of all the scar tissue in an injured area, but instead to create the most functional scar possible. A functional scar is one that allows a certain degree of mobility to the injured tissue, similar to the degree of mobility that was present in the original uninjured tissue. The same time that mobility is offered, the scar will prevent excessive stress from causing a recurrence or aggravation of the injury.

2. Neurological Dysfunction

The second category of conditions that contribute to orthopedic disorders are those that involve neurological dysfunction. Many massage practitioners do not get taught a comprehensive model of the neurological system. This leaves a great deal of territory open for misinterpretation and confusion when trying to determine how to work with various clients. Problems that involve neurological dysfunction may take many different forms. We will investigate some of those variations in the following sections.

In a very simplified model, the neurological system can be thought of as a central information processing station (central nervous system) with relay lines sending signals to the distant parts, and bringing signals back to the central processing station. The lines that send signals away from the central processing station and bring them back would be analogous to the peripheral nervous system. Signals that go away from the central nervous system (CNS), known as efferent signals, will carry messages that cause certain actions to happen to remote tissues. An example is the signal that is sent to a muscle causing it to contract. Signals that report from the peripheral nervous system (PNS) back to the CNS will provide many different types of sensory information such as pressure, temperature, pain, or position in space. For example, during the course of a massage treatment your CNS is receiving many different signals about levels of pain, pressure, or texture on your skin that are being processed (usually) as a pleasurable sensation. There are some treatment methods, such as deep transverse friction massage, which may perceived as an uncomfortable or even painful sensation. By remembering the types of information carried by the neurological system, an aware practitioner can determine different levels of involvement by neurological structures.

In the course of assessment there are several sensations the massage practitioner is encouraged to become aware of. Each of these different sensations may give a different clue as to what is happening in the tissues. Pain is a primary neurological sensation to be aware of. Although pain obviously does not always indicate neurological involvement, there are certain descriptions of pain that should flag the practitioner's awareness that neurological structures might be involved. Pain that a client reports as searing, burning, shooting, or electrical in nature should tip off the practitioner that neurological structures may be involved. This may be compression of a nerve trunk, nerve root, or stretching of a nerve.

Paresthesia (pins and needles sensations) is another descriptive category to be aware of. Paresthesia is usually caused by compression on a nerve somewhere along its path. However, as with many conditions that have neurological involvement, paresthesia can be tricky. In many instances the sensation of pins and needles tends to come on when the pressure has been released. An example is when you get up from a sitting position where you had your legs crossed for several minutes. As you start to walk across the floor, a shower of pins and needles sensations overtakes you. It is usually not immediate but happens shortly after the compression has been released.

Another interesting factor of nerve compression and paresthesia is something Dr. James Cyriax, the British Orthopedic Physician, described relating to this compression-release phenomenon. In describing how the sensation of paresthesia appears to come about after release of the compression, he also noted that the duration of the compression was an important factor in determining when the paresthesia began. For example, if you compressed the peroneal nerve in your leg by crossing your legs for five minutes and then got up and walked on it, you would feel the sensation of paresthesia less than a minute after having released it. However, if that nerve had been compressed all day, such as the nerves of the brachial plexus often are when pressed against the upper rib cage, you might not release that compression until you went to bed at night and rolled over on you side. The sensation of paresthesia may not come about for several hours. People will often describe waking up several hours after going to bed with their arms "asleep" or "numb". This description may lead you to look for possible brachial plexus compression.

Another neurological sensation is numbness. Since the neurological system is transmitting sensory information to the brain, impairment of function in the neurological system is likely to interrupt the transmission of these signals. Numbness is caused by a lack of sensory signals being transmitted to the brain. There is no sensation of pressure, temperature, texture, etc. Of course the impairment may not be complete and those signals might be only slightly impaired and not cut off completely. In either event, the client is likely to report numbness if the sensation is impaired.

The above descriptions of neurological impairment all involve afferent or sensory signals. Efferent signals may be disrupted from conditions with neurological involvement as well. Efferent signals, for example, are responsible for giving a contraction stimulus to the muscles. The degree of contraction in the muscles may depend on the amount of stimulus that the neurological system will transmit. If there is an impairment to neurological signals, the receiving station (muscles in this case) will not perform to their full capability. This may show up as muscle weakness, atrophy, or in a severe case as paralysis. When muscles do not get an adequate contraction stimulus, the biomechanical balance around the joint will be upset. This biomechanical imbalance will lead to further soft-tissue distress. A cycle of impairment and dysfunction is then likely to develop.

An aspect of neurological dysfunction that has received a great deal of attention in the massage profession is that of referred pain. Referred pain or other referred sensations are the result of improper neurological function. When there is too much neurological input from an area, there is a signal processing error that happens within the brain. The brain perceives pain as originating from an area that is not where the faulty tissue is located. A common example of this phenomenon is a myofascial trigger point. A local area of hyperirritability may develop in a muscle. When that area is subjected to additional stress (contraction, stretch, or direct compression for example), signals will be sent back to the brain, but will be perceived as originating from some other remote location. Therefore a myofascial trigger point located in the neck may cause a pain to be felt in the temporal region of the head.

The treatment of myofascial trigger points with massage has gotten a great deal of attention in the last several years. This is one type of neurological dysfunction which is best treated with correctly applied massage therapy (which may include stretching methods such as muscle energy technique). A knowledge of anatomy, muscle function, basic neurological concepts, and trigger point referral patterns will be important in making this type of treatment effective. Trigger points may develop in any muscle at any time. The referred pain sensations can become very confusing when trying to determine the nature of soft-tissue pain and where it is originating. Again, this stresses the importance of thorough assessment. The more you are able to understand about the nature of these types of problems, the better you will be at determining if there is referred pain involved or if it is a local tissue that is creating the problem. The reader interested in learning more about myofascial trigger points is encouraged to study the works of Janet Travell, M.D. and David Simons, M.D. (see reference section).

Psychogenic pain, a pain sensation with a strong psychological component deserves mention here. It is included with the discussion of neurological dysfunction because it most closely resembles problems that involve signal transmission through the neurological system. Pain has a psychological component, but what distinguishes psychogenic pain is that the psychological component appears to be a *primary* factor in the perpetuation of the pain. Psychogenic pain has been a particularly controversial topic for many health care practitioners. Most of that controversy is rooted in conflicting models and paradigms of how the body functions. At the present time we still don't have a great deal of hard evidence to support any one particular theory about the nature of psychogenic pain. However, anyone who has spent time practicing therapeutic massage will certainly tell you that this is a very real phenomena that many clients encounter.

Psychogenic pain may take several different forms. A simple example is looking at how pain is perceived by different people. There are numerous factors, many of them psychologically influenced, which may affect how pain is perceived. These factors include social structure and environment, ethnic background, corresponding levels of stress, and personal psychological make up. What is a severe pain for one person is only a mild discomfort for someone else. A person may also talk themselves "out of" or "in to" pain. For example, if a competitive athlete is in the middle of the performance of a lifetime, he or she may be able to psychologically override many different pain sensations. Conversely, a person who is trying to avoid work or something unpleasant may perceive their pain as being increasingly severe.

One of the most interesting aspects of psychogenic pain is that which is associated with psychological memory. In order to understand this, you must transcend the barriers between different systems which study human function. It is interesting to note that traditional Western medical science has stayed very clear of psychological elements when studying their patient's pathologies. Yet common sense tells us that our psychological experiences are an integral part of our physiology. We may smell something that immediately brings us back to a memory from our distant past. That memory will call up emotions, visual images, or kinesthetic (tactile) sensations. All of these different components appeared to be triggered by the smell. It appears that each of our senses can cause that same trigger phenomenon to occur, and it will often occur when we least expect it. Because of the powerful stimuli that the body receives during massage therapy, especially the tactile and kinesthetic stimuli, certain memories or experiences which have been very deep below the level of conscious awareness may surface. This will often happen quite unexpectedly for the client. These "psychological" memories may involve pain sensations that are being "remembered" by the neurological receptors.

The problem in trying to define psychogenic pain comes in trying to apply a mechanical model (which is usually the dominant method of analysis in Western medicine) to these situations. It is unlikely that you will be able to come up with any consistent explanation for the pain that the client experiences. It is in many of these situations that a person is told by some health care practitioner that "...it's all in your head". Since it is the brain that perceives pain there may be some truth in that statement. However, that does not make the pain any less real. When performing assessment of orthopedic problems it is crucial to remember that the psychological component can't be removed from the equation in determining the true nature of your client's condition. Again, this is another wonderful benefit that massage practitioners may offer. The nature of massage therapy is such that the client can be addressed on a multidimensional level. The massage practitioner can treat mechanical problems of the body structure while encouraging a positive psychological environment. This will enhance the healing potential for psychological components of the client's problem.

How to use assessment procedures.

Analysis of the different ways in which the body can become injured is valuable as an academic exercise, but how can it help the clinical practitioner? One of the most important aspects of learning to use assessment procedures is developing the skills and knowledge to:

match the physiology of the tissue injury
with the
physiological effects of specific treatment methods

This means that the practitioner will pay attention to what caused the pain or injury and then select the most appropriate treatment approach. For example, if a pain condition is primarily caused by muscular tightness and myofascial trigger points, the most appropriate treatment will probably include static compression or methods that decrease neurological activity and enhance muscle elongation. Longitudinal stripping strokes and stretching would work well for this purpose. A technique, such as deep transverse friction massage, designed to break up fibrous scar tissue would not be best here, and in some instances may aggravate the problem.

The analysis of problems and selection of treatments sounds simple, but many clinical practitioners do not go through this process. As a result their treatments are much less effective. It is important to remember that many problems may be a complex blend of mechanical tissue disruption and excessive neurological activity. Therefore, some combination of methods will get the best results. The art of the skilled practitioner is being able to choose the most appropriate method and make certain that it fits for each unique situation that the individual client will present.

CHAPTER 2

THE SOFT-TISSUES: DEFINITIONS, ROLES, AND DYSFUNCTIONS

This chapter will focus on the function of the soft-tissues and how they respond to a variety of stresses. A helpful classification of these tissues is that compiled by Dr. James Cyriax (Cyriax 1982). He classifies the soft tissues as either contractile or inert. The contractile tissues are those which are actively engaged in a contraction process in order to create movement in the body. This includes muscles and tendons. Even though a tendon does not generate a contraction within its own fibers, it is considered a contractile tissue because of its function in transmitting the contraction force of a muscle to the bone.

The inert tissues include joint capsule, ligament, bursa, fascia, dura mater and nerve. There are other soft tissue structures of the body which are not included here such as vascular structures and organs. The purpose of this classification is to focus on those tissues which are most involved with creating and limiting movement in the body. We will look at each of these tissues, their function, and ways in which they are injured.

MUSCLE

Muscle is the primary contractile tissue. It has an important role in maintaining posture, creating movement, slowing or stopping movement, and giving us sensory feedback about our position in space and contact with the outside world. Individual fibers in the muscle which are wrapped in bundles will actively contract when stimulated by a nerve impulse. When that nerve impulse ceases, the muscle will cease the contraction. Contractions often perpetuate because of excess signals that are unnecessary. The interested student is encouraged to review the complex physiological process that is involved with muscular contraction in more detail in an appropriate physiology text.

It is helpful to understand what role the muscle is playing in a particular movement or activity. This is essential during the assessment process and will greatly assist the practitioner in making recommendations about treatment and home care or work suggestions for the client. Muscle function can be divided into four separate categories listed below. The function that a muscle will have is dependent on the movement which is being examined. For example in one movement a muscle will be an agonist or prime mover, when in another movement that same muscle will be an antagonist. The practitioner must examine the movement to determine what role that muscle is playing.

Agonist or prime mover- is a muscle which is responsible for creating a particular movement. For example, we would say that the quadriceps muscle group is a prime mover for knee extension against resistance. As you will see in the next section, it is not clear enough to say simply that the quadriceps are the prime mover for knee extension. There are certain situations in which knee extension may be occurring, but the quadriceps are not involved in creating this movement. This will be explained in the section below dealing with eccentric muscle contractions.

Fixator or stabilizer- is a muscle which is supporting or holding some body part steady so that other muscles attached to that part may engage in contraction. An example is the rhomboid muscles which often act as stabilizers of the scapula during arm movements. They contract to hold the scapula steady so that some of the other muscles which attach to the scapula and move the arm may be more effective in creating the desired movement. As a fixator, a muscle may be attempting to hold a body part still in relation to the forces of gravity acting on the body. An example of this is the erector spinae muscle group on the side of the spine which contracts in order to fixate or stabilize the spine in an upright position while we are standing, sitting, or walking.

Neutralizer- is a muscle which is engaged to prevent an undesirable action of another muscle. For example, if the desired action was extension of the arm, the teres major muscle would be utilized as a prime mover or agonist. However, the teres major also medially rotates the arm and medial rotation of the arm is not desired for this particular movement. For that reason the infraspinatus, a lateral rotator, would be called upon to resist or "neutralize" the medial rotation so that only extension was produced. This is an oversimplified description of how movement actually occurs, but it will help to see how the muscles are working in conjunction with each other while performing various different roles. This also illustrates how difficult it is to fully isolate one muscle's action when testing any movement.

Antagonist- is a muscle whose action is opposite that of an agonist or prime mover is referred to as the antagonist. In extension of the knee against resistance, the quadriceps will be the prime mover and the hamstrings will be antagonists. Understanding the sometimes complex agonist/antagonist relationships will be an important component in helping to analyze movement and determine which tissues are at fault. It will also be an important part of giving home care suggestions to a client which might involve stretching or strengthening activities.

The literature on muscle function and contraction is often confusing because the terms which are used are not fully defined and sometimes used inappropriately. A full discussion of types of muscle contraction is beyond the scope of this book, but we will define several terms which will be used when discussing muscle contraction.

Concentric contraction- is one in which the muscle's two ends are brought closer together and the muscle shortens during the active contraction phase. An example of a concentric contraction in the biceps brachii muscle is the upward lifting phase of a "curl" where the arm is flexing at the elbow and the wrist is being brought toward the shoulder while raising a weight. In strength training this movement is also called "positive" work of the muscle. Concentric contractions are relatively easy to identify if you are familiar with muscle actions for that particular muscle. They are associated with acceleration movements of the body. When a muscle action is listed in an anatomy or physiology text, they will be listing the concentric contraction of that muscle.

Isometric contraction- is one in which no movement is produced at the joint despite the active contraction in the muscle. If an outside resistance (our weight in the above biceps curl example for instance) equally matches the amount of contraction stimulus in the muscle and the weight is held still, then no movement will be produced at the joint. If you go halfway down into a deep knee bend and hold it there you are engaging in many isometric contractions when you get to the point of holding the deep knee bend position. The contractions in your muscles which are resisting the pull of gravity are not lifting you up, they are only holding you in the half-bent position. Therefore no movement is occurring at your joints. This is an isometric contraction. Isometric contractions are used by muscles in their role as stabilizers

Eccentric contraction- An eccentric contraction seems somewhat like a contradiction in terms because it is a contraction in which the muscle actually elongates. There is a nerve stimulus to the muscle which is exciting its fibers, but the outside resistance is greater than the intensity of the stimulus to the muscle. Therefore the outside resistance overcomes the muscle's "attempt to contract". During an eccentric contraction the muscle is being stimulated to contract, but it is getting longer. In strength training this movement is commonly referred to as "negative" work. Using our example of the biceps brachii, when the weight that is raised up to the shoulder during the concentric phase is slowly lowered back down to the beginning position, an eccentric contraction is happening in that muscle.

NOTE: As long as the speed of its return is slower than the speed that gravity would naturally cause it to return, there will be an eccentric contraction. If the return is done simply by letting the arm go limp, it is actually gravity that does the work. In this instance there is a passive elongation of the biceps and a passive shortening of the triceps. If the weight is rapidly and forcefully returned to the beginning position (faster than gravity would allow it to fall), then the biceps brachii is no longer involved in creating the movement. It is the triceps which has created the movement. In each of these three situations there is the same motion (extension) happening at the elbow. However, what produces that extension is different for each of the three different situations. This is why it is not sufficient to say that the triceps muscle produces elbow extension as a blanket statement. What produces elbow extension is dependent on numerous other factors of motion which must be taken into consideration. This may seem overly technical, but it is a crucial part of analyzing how muscles are playing a role in an injury condition.

Eccentric muscle contractions are most often used when decelerating movement or resisting gravity (a special type of deceleration). It is sometimes harder to distinguish eccentric muscle contractions because many people are accustomed to thinking that if a muscle is lengthening, then it must be passively stretching and not contracting.

A thorough understanding of these types of muscle contractions is crucial to the performance of effective rehabilitative massage. One of the best ways to really understand muscle contractions is to take simple actions of the body and see if you can determine what types of muscle contractions are happening with those movements.

A great deal of attention is placed on muscle contractions but an equally important part of muscle function is the muscle's ability to elongate. Muscle tissue has the property of extensibility which means that it can be stretched in addition to being able to contract. In fact, a great limiting factor to how effective a muscle contraction will be is the level of extensibility of that muscle. A muscle which remains in a shortened position for a long time is likely to become dysfunctional. It may become weak or develop fibrous tissue that limits its ability to elongate. This is called a contracture. If a muscle is limited in its ability to elongate, we say that muscle is tight or the person is inflexible in that particular area. As we look at ideal muscle balance and biomechanical function around the joints, the importance of a strength/ flexibility equilibrium will become apparent.

The most common type of acute injury to muscles is a tensile stress injury in which fibers are disrupted because their two ends are being pulled beyond the muscle's extensibility. This same mechanism of injury may also be present in certain chronic muscle injuries. This is why muscle injuries of this type are often called a "pulled" muscle. The correct term for this injury is a strain. Muscle strains are divided into three grades in order to clarify their severity. They are as follows:

First Degree or Grade 1 Strain- is a mild strain. There has been some disruption of muscle fibers. It is unlikely that there will be pain with active movement of the body part without resistance. There may be some pain associated with active movement against resistance. There may also be some mild degree of pain associated with the very end range of motion when the muscle is stretched. It is not likely that there will be any palpable defect with a grade 1 strain. The palpable defect is a clearly palpable area where the fibers have been disrupted.

Second Degree or Grade 2 Strain- is a moderate strain. A greater number of fibers have been torn than with the grade 1 strain, and there is likely to be pain with active motion even without any external resistance. Active contraction against resistance will usually cause pain, as will stretching the affected area. Depending on the severity of the strain, a palpable defect may be present in a grade 2 strain. The palpable defect is also likely to be tender or painful. There will almost certainly be limitation to function as a result of this strain.

Third Degree or Grade 3 Strain- is a severe strain or complete rupture of the muscle tendon unit. There will likely be severe pain associated with the immediate onset of this condition. There will be significant impairment and may be complete loss of function. However, the presence of some function does not mean that a grade 3 strain is not present. Other muscles may be compensating or assisting in the movement. Any resisted movements will be weak if at all present, but may not be severely painful due to injury of the nerve fibers in the area. If the muscle tendon unit is not completely ruptured there will be a significant palpable defect. A grade 3 strain will often produce ecchymosis (bruising) which may appear to get worse several days after the actual injury. A grade 3 strain may be left untreated in certain conditions. When it heals there will be a noticeable divot in the continuity of the muscle.

One of the most common ways that muscles are strained is through excessive eccentric loading. In the previous section eccentric muscle contractions were described. When a muscle is having to work eccentrically against a significant resistance, there is a greater likelihood that a strain will occur. A muscle is capable of handling heavier loads eccentrically, but there are fewer fibers being recruited. It is this heavy eccentric loading that overwhelms the muscle fibers and causes them to tear. This may happen because the tensile strength of the tendon is so great. The tendon is much more resistant to tensile stress than the muscle is and therefore it is often the muscle fibers which end up being damaged. This will overwhelm them causing a strain.

Another type of acute injury that muscles may be subjected to involves compression stress to the muscle which disrupts its fibers. This is called a contusion. A contusion will often happen in contact sports or traumatic accidents such as automobile wrecks. When a muscle is injured from a contusion it will undergo a healing process which will attempt to repair the injured area and any disrupted fibers.

There is a neurological patterning or "memory" that your muscle tissues have which may cause them to hold a significant amount of tension following a traumatic incident such as a contusion. This may lead to an excessive amount of unnecessary contraction by the muscle which will eventually cause further imbalances and dysfunction.

Muscle spasm is one of the most common types of dysfunction or "injury" that is present in the human body. It may be quite severe and debilitating, as in the case of a muscle cramp, or it may be only mildly or occasionally irritating. In any event, this is a condition which is impairing optimal function, and which will respond quite well to rehabilitative massage.

Excessive neurological activity in a muscle will cause that muscle to contract more than is actually necessary. This excessive activity may be caused by numerous factors. Previous injuries, improper biomechanics, emotional trauma, stress- all these can play a role in creating chronic tension in the muscles. We have very little control over how those muscles choose to store the tension. The increased amount of tension in the muscles will interfere with their proper coordinated function. If for no other reason, this is one of the best reasons to utilize rehabilitative massage treatment. Massage is very effective in reducing unnecessary muscular tension.

Myofascial trigger points are a unique phenomena that greatly effect the proper functioning of muscles. The exhaustive clinical research of Janet Travell & David Simons (Travell & Simons, 1983, 1992) has done a tremendous amount to advance our understanding of trigger point phenomena in the body. Trigger points are areas of hyperirritability in the muscle tissue which may refer pain or other sensations to a remote area. A practitioner may press on a trigger point in the neck, for example, and the client will feel a sharp pain around the side of the head. There is not a muscle that traverses that exact path, so something else is going on.

There is still a great deal to be learned about trigger points. They seem to be caused by an error in perception on the part of the brain as to where the offending tissue is located. For instance, in our earlier example of the trigger point, the brain perceives the problem to be around the side of the head instead of in the neck. Myofascial trigger points are a phenomena that must be looked at as a neuromuscular condition - meaning one that involves both the muscular system and the neurological system.

TENDON

The primary role of tendon tissue is to transmit the contractile force of the muscle to the bone in order to move the bone. For this reason tendons are relatively inflexible structures which are designed to be strongest in the direction of tensile stress. Most of the fibers of a tendon will run in a longitudinal direction in the tendon. This will give it the greatest amount of tensile strength. Figure 2-1 shows the fiber orientation of a tendon.

Figure 2-1
*Fiber orientation of a tendon.
Notice the parallel direction
of fibers which give a tendon
its great tensile strength.*

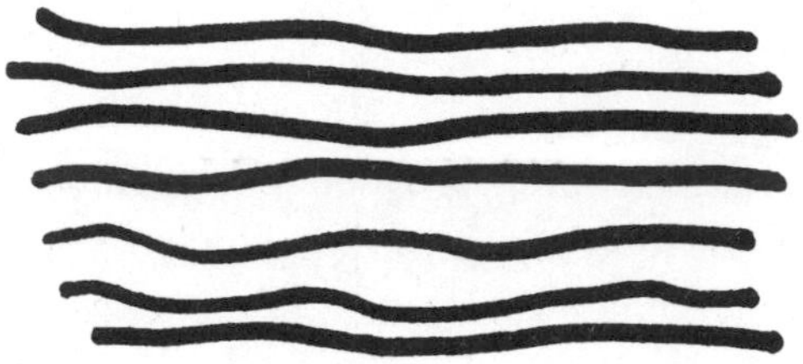

Tendons do not contract but they are considered part of the group of tissues known as contractile tissues because they function so interdependently with muscle. For that reason we often speak of the muscle/tendon unit as a whole.

Despite their great strength, tendons are most susceptible to excessive tensile stress injuries. However, the way in which tendons develop tensile stress injuries is usually different than how they occur to muscles. Muscle strains occur most often with heavy eccentric loading. Tensile stress injuries occur to tendons in one of two common ways - sudden forceful loading and chronic sub-maximal loading.

Luckily, complete tendon tears, also known as a rupture, are infrequent. They are painful, debilitating and will usually require surgical repair. It has been estimated that most tendons are only exposed to about 25% of the tensile stress that they are capable of handling during normal daily movement. Because the tendon is so resistant to tensile stress it takes a great deal of force to rupture a tendon.

There are, however, a few tendons which are particularly vulnerable to the types of stress that may cause a rupture. The most commonly ruptured tendon is the Achilles tendon. This often happens with jumping athletes. The individual will usually have tight calf muscles (gastrocnemius & soleus, also known as the triceps surae) to start with. When that person jumps up, the triceps surae contracts concentrically. They may still be engaged in a contraction stimulus when the person's toes hit the ground a few seconds later. When the toes hit the ground the triceps surae is immediately engaged in an eccentric contraction. This may so overwhelm the tensile strength of the tendon that it will rupture as a result.

A more frequent tendon injury involves what is known as repetitive sub-maximal loading. A tendon is subjected to a force which is well within its physiological limits, but it is subjected to that force over and over again. This does not completely overwhelm the tendon as a whole but the fibers of the tendon do suffer from stress fatigue. This causes small micro-tearing of the tendon fibers. This is the cause of tendinitis. Often the microtearing will occur at an area of poor mechanical strength such as the musculotendinous junction. Ceasing the offending movement is generally the best method of treating tendinitis, but that method has subsequent problems which will be discussed later.

Another type of overuse injury which affects tendons is tenosynovitis. Tenosynovitis is often confused with tendinitis, but the cause of the problem is quite different. Certain tendons, especially those around the distal extremities, have to make significant bends in their path. It is difficult for the tendon to effectively deliver the contraction force of the muscle to its bony attachment when the tendon has to take a curve. For that reason there is a soft-tissue structure, often a retinaculum (a binding soft tissue band or restraint) which will hold the tendon close to the joint. In order to reduce friction on the tendon, these tendons are surrounded by a sheath which acts like a protective sleeve.

If there is excessive pressure or irritation between a tendon and its sheath, the tendon surface will begin to roughen slightly and may eventually form fibrous adhesions to the sheath. This will prevent effective gliding of the tendon within the sheath. Movement that happens with this condition will frequently have crepitus, a subtle grinding sensation which can be felt or possibly heard. It is important to remember that not all tendons have sheaths. It is mainly the ones associated with the distal extremities. Most anatomy texts will give a good distinction for which tendons do and do not have sheaths.

An additional tensile stress injury will be mentioned here even though it primarily involves the bone where the tendon inserts. This is called a tendon avulsion or avulsion fracture. If a tendon is subjected to a high degree of tensile stress it may tear or rupture. In certain cases the tendon will remain intact, but will tear away from its attachment at the bone. It also may tear away a small chunk of bone with it. Figure 2-2 depicts an avulsion fracture.

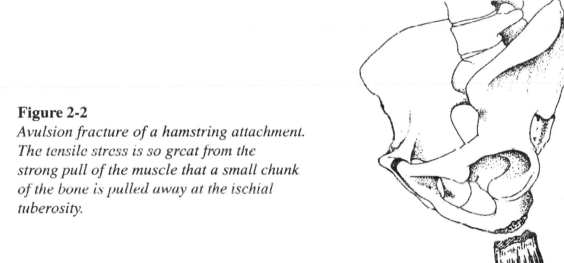

Figure 2-2
Avulsion fracture of a hamstring attachment. The tensile stress is so great from the strong pull of the muscle that a small chunk of the bone is pulled away at the ischial tuberosity.

Depending on its severity and the distance that the tendon has pulled away from the bone, it may need surgical repair. No matter how severe this condition is, it is likely to be very painful because the periosteum of the bone where the tendon inserts is a very pain sensitive tissue.

LIGAMENTS

The primary function of ligamentous tissue is to create stability around the joints. Ligaments connect adjacent bones to each other and help to prevent excessive movement in specific planes relative to that joint. There are more transverse fibers in ligamentous tissue than in tendon tissue. This allows the ligament to be more resistant to stress in multiple directions. The tendon only encounters tensile stress along its length from muscle contraction. The ligament is designed to be strong in one predominant direction (the line of tensile stress along its length), but also must be resistant to multidirectional stresses that the joint may encounter during movement.

Figure 2-3
Orientation of ligament fibers.
The parallel arrangement of ligament
fibers is complemented by some fibers
which cross in a transverse direction.
This gives the ligament an ability
to resist stress in several different
planes.

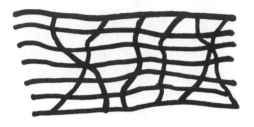

Ligament also has a greater concentration of elastin than the tendon does. This will allow the ligament a small degree of "give" before it pulls taut at that particular joint. This small amount of "give" is important. If the ligament were as rigid and "ungiving" to tensile stress as a tendon, the frequency of ligament injuries would be much greater.

The most common injury to a ligament is an excessive tensile stress injury. Similar to muscle strains, ligament sprains are categorized and graded on a scale which divides the severity of the injury into three categories. Injury to the muscle tendon unit is called a strain. Injury to the ligamentous tissue is called a sprain.

First Degree or Grade 1 Sprain- is a mild sprain will be characterized by some stretching or tearing of ligamentous fibers. There may be some slight pain on active or passive motion of that joint. Joint stability will generally not be hindered. Swelling and joint stiffness are also likely to accompany the sprain.

Second Degree or Grade 2 Sprain- is a moderate sprain will have a greater number of fibers disrupted. Swelling and pain may be moderate to severe. Joint stiffness following the injury is likely to set in some hours later. A grade 2 sprain will also cause some joint instability.

Third Degree or Grade 3 Sprain- is a severe or total rupture of the ligament and will be characterized by a great deal of instability around the joint. The client may describe a sensation that the joint is going to "give way" if any weight is put on it. This injury will be painful at the immediate onset, but may not cause significant pain later due to the rupture of neurological fibers in the area. Swelling is likely to be extensive and will limit mobility around the joint. As a result of the trauma associated with the sprain, local muscles that cross the joint are also likely to go into spasm in an attempt to prevent excessive movement at the joint. This is important to remember when testing the integrity of ligament structures or mobility at a joint because a severe ligament injury may not seem as bad if the muscles surrounding the joint are in enough spasm to prevent certain movements. To produce enough force to create a grade 3 ligament sprain other surrounding tissues will often be injured.

JOINT CAPSULE

The composition of joint capsule tissue is similar to that of ligament tissue. Its primary function is to maintain integrity of the joint, guide specific joint motions, prevent excessive motion, and house the lubricating synovial fluid which reduces friction and wear on the joints. Portions of the joint capsule are highly innervated with proprioceptors and nociceptors. Proprioceptors are specialized cells that give a great deal of feedback information to the central nervous system about movement and position in space. Nociceptors are pain receptors. Injuries to the joint capsule may be quite painful. The most common types of injuries sustained by the joint capsule are tensile stress tearing injuries such as those sustained by ligaments. However capsular tears are not graded in the three grades as ligament injuries are.

The joint capsule also may be involved in various conditions of adhesion that will limit functional range of motion. For numerous reasons, some of them unknown, a joint capsule will begin to develop adhesions and restrictions to movement in certain planes of motion. This may involve muscle spasm and tightness, prolonged immobilization, repetitive misuse, or emotional factors. The condition of adhesive capsulitis, also known as frozen shoulder, is an example of this. We don't often think of applying massage for conditions of capsular adhesion because it is usually very difficult to directly palpate the joint capsule. However, many of the methods of rehabilitative massage will be quite helpful in managing problems with adhered joint capsules.

CARTILAGE

There are two types of cartilage that will be of primary concern with locomotor disorders: hyaline cartilage and fibrocartilage. This cartilage does not have vascular or nerve supply. This is important because injury to the actual cartilage tissue may not feel painful to the individual. Many times it is only when the injured cartilage interferes with some other type of tissue that pain or discomfort will be felt.

Hyaline cartilage is prominent at the ends of the bones in joints where it is called articular cartilage. It is a hard, shiny substance which greatly reduces friction on the bones and helps to create a smooth gliding surface for the two ends of the bone that are meeting. Fibrocartilage is also present between the bones but it plays a different role. Fibrocartilage can be found in regions such as the menisci of the knee or the intervertebral disks in the spine. These fibrocartilage "disks" in both the knee and the spine help to provide additional cushioning from compressive forces. The intervertebral disks also help to angle the spine and the menisci in the knee help to provide the optimum contact surfaces required for functional joint mechanics.

Cartilage is susceptible to several types of injuries. Compressive force injuries to cartilage are the most frequent. Disk herniations and ruptures of the intervertebral disks in the spine are a result of cumulative compressive forces over time. They may be made suddenly worse by an acute injury, but there is usually a history of chronic compression needed to fully herniate or rupture a disk.

The menisci in the knee or articular cartilage in any of the weight-bearing joints may be subject to cracking or splitting from excessive compressive forces over time. When we run, for example, we put compressive forces on our weight bearing joints of the lower extremity that are 3 to 4 times our body weight.

There are not many tensile stress injuries which happen to cartilage structures because it is actually quite difficult to put tensile stress on most of them. One exception is the medial meniscus of the knee. There are fibers of the medial (tibial) collateral ligament of the knee which are also attached to the medial meniscus. For that reason, if the medial collateral ligament is severely sprained, as in a serious and sudden valgus stress to the knee, portions of the meniscus may be torn as a result. A valgus stress is one that puts a force on the lateral side of the knee and is aimed in a medial direction.

Applications of massage will not be aimed at directly affecting these cartilage structures. Most of them will not be palpable. However many other factors such as compensating muscular balance and altered soft-tissue mechanics will result from cartilage injuries. Rehabilitative massage approaches may have beneficial effects on these other structures, thereby indirectly helping the cartilage injury to heal. In addition, it may be an imbalance of muscular forces around a joint that is causing the chronic compression on a cartilage structure. Massage may be helpful in relieving that chronic compressive force.

FASCIA

It seems that medical literature of the not so recent past almost ignored the importance of fascia. Now it is getting quite a lot of attention, especially with those practitioners who spend a great deal of time with soft-tissue injuries. Fascia is the complex soft-tissue webbing which holds us all together. It is: wrapped around muscles, wrapped around individual muscle fibers, used in suspending organs, a necessary matrix for vascular structures, nerves, and lymphatic vessels, and instrumental in creating our body shape.

Fascia is a connective tissue and therefore its tensile strength is very important. It is quite pliable and malleable so it is rarely subjected to compressive force injuries. The main problems with fascia are tensile stress injuries and the problematic results created from periods of prolonged shortening.

When soft tissue structures of the body are overstretched, the fascia that binds or connects them will also be overstretched. The fascia has multidirectional fibers in order to resist stress from different directions. However, if that stress overcomes the tensile strength of the fascia, it will tear. When it does, it is likely to create scar tissue which may bind the fascia to adjacent structures. This scar tissue is most easily managed during the rehabilitation process by multi directional stress (massage strokes, stretching, etc.) being applied to it within its comfortable and normal range of motion.

One of the most problematic features of fascia is its response to prolonged immobilization. If the body is held in one position for long periods of time the fascia has a tendency to adapt to that position. This is especially problematic when the fascia is held in a shortened position. When it is kept in this shortened position, it will structurally adapt to that position and resist an attempt to return to its normal length. The longer it is subjected to this shortening, the harder it will be for it to return to its normal length.

A common example is for someone who has an injured clavicle and must hold their arm in a sling with the elbow bent to about 90 degrees of flexion. When they finally take their arm out of the sling, the clavicle injury may be well on its way to healing, but they have developed flexion contractures, or fascial binding in the elbow flexor muscles from a chronic shortening of the fascia. Here is an example of how massage may not be aimed at the primary injury (the clavicle) but may in fact be highly useful in managing a secondary condition which developed as a result of the first.

NERVE

The communication and function of the nervous system is a vast and complex subject. Entire textbooks are written on it and we are still learning how the nervous system functions. Major nerve trunks carry signals that are going in two directions. The afferent signals are the incoming signals from the periphery of the nervous system back to the central processing centers, the brain and spinal cord. These afferent signals are the sensory information that we are taking in from the outside world. The efferent signals are the outgoing impulses which are specifically encoded to cause some action at the far end of the nerve receptor such as a muscle contraction. The signal for the muscle contraction starts in the brain and ends in the electrochemical process of muscle contraction that produces the desired movement. It should be obvious even from this simplistic representation that we rely heavily on the effective functioning of our nervous system. It is our communication network and it is essential for our survival.

We often think of the nerves as long thin channels which transmit the signal impulses. Because the primary functions of nerve tissue are electrochemical in nature and not mechanical, they are not resilient to various forms of mechanical stress such as compression or tension. Nerve tissue may be injured from compressive force injuries. These injuries may be either acute or chronic. An example of an acute nerve compression injury is where you suddenly compress the ulnar nerve at the elbow (the "funny bone"). There is an immediate onslaught of neurological reporting from this compression force. Your hand or forearm may hurt, burn, or tingle for several minutes following the injury. If the injury is severe enough, these sensations will persist for much longer. A much more severe compression could cause temporary or permanent paralysis.

A common example of a chronic compressive force injury is carpal tunnel syndrome. Improper mechanics of the hand and swelling of the flexor tendons of the hand cause a narrowing of the channel in the carpal tunnel. The median nerve is then constantly compressed causing pain, paresthesia (pins and needles sensations), numbness, or possible loss of function. The variety of responses to compression injuries can be quite varied.

An interesting phenomenon is described by James Cyriax (Cyriax 1982) regarding nerve compression. He describes situations in which the pain and discomfort from nerve compression are felt not upon the compression, but after the fact when compression is released. Interesting information about the location of the compression may also be gained from the types of sensations that the client is reporting. For example, pressure on the distal portion of a nerve may be more likely to produce pain and numbness, whereas pressure on the proximal region of the nerve will be more likely to produce sensations of paresthesia.

Nerve tissue is also quite susceptible to tensile stress injuries. These are most often associated with an acute or sudden elongating of the nerve trunk. An example of this condition is the injury called a cervical burner or stinger. This is an injury that happens as a result of a sudden and forceful lateral flexion of the neck to one side. The brachial plexus on the opposite side will then be suddenly elongated past the point of natural elasticity of the nerve tissue. This will produce symptoms similar to the compressive force injuries such as pain, paresthesia, numbness, and possible loss of function in the areas supplied by the nerves that were injured. Depending on the severity of the stretch of the nerve tissue, these symptoms will persist for varied amounts of time.

Massage applications directly to the involved nerve tissue in compressive or tensile stress injuries are not likely to be helpful. This is because they are likely to cause more discomfort than they will alleviate. However, surrounding musculature may have gone into a protective spasm that is exacerbating the symptoms and the primary problem. Or, as in the case of carpal tunnel syndrome, it is the tightness of the muscles that is a contributing factor to the development of the condition. So again, the application of rehabilitative massage will be geared toward contributing through an indirect effect more than a direct effect on the involved nerve tissue.

BURSA

The bursa is a small fluid-filled sac that provides cushioning and reduces friction in joints and areas of high friction in the body. The bursa will act as a buffer between certain structures to keep them from rubbing on and irritating each other. Because of its role as a friction reducer, the bursae are most subject to compressive force injuries. They may be either chronic or acute. The most common types of compression injuries to bursae are chronic injuries which cause the bursa to become inflamed. This is the condition of bursitis.

Bursitis is most common as an overuse syndrome where there is one particular motion which is repeated over and over again such as the common shoulder bursitis experienced by swimmers from repetitive overhead motions of the arm. Bursitis in certain regions may cause a *painful arc,* which is evident during evaluation movements. A painful arc is a portion of a certain movement which causes pain. There will usually not be pain in the early phase of movement, the pain will then come on for a certain "arc" of that movement, and then cease after a certain point. For example, if the shoulder were moving in a straight frontal plane abduction movement, the client could move pain free until about 45° of abduction. At 45° the pain would begin and they would feel pain all the way through about 130° of abduction. After that point the pain would cease. The region between 45° and 130° is considered to be the painful arc.

For bursitis and other compression injuries to the bursa, the most effective massage applications will not be administered directly to the injured bursa. The best benefits can be derived from applications to the associated tissues which are involved with the compression. A working knowledge of functional anatomy and kinesiology will be helpful in recommending modifications of mechanics to the client for the activities which are causing the problem.

This overview of the structure, function, and common injury methods of the contractile and inert tissues will provide the framework for understanding what happens with the specific conditions mentioned later in the book. Now that the nature of various tissue injuries has been introduced, we will turn our attention to how we can put this information into a useful format. One of the most comprehensive and effective methods of assessment is the HOPS procedure that is commonly used in orthopedics and sports medicine. In the next chapter we will outline the HOPS method of assessment and discuss how it can be applied to the massage therapy environment.

CHAPTER 3

THE H.O.P.S. METHOD OF SOFT-TISSUE ASSESSMENT

There are many different ways to approach soft-tissue assessment. Most practitioners will find they get the best results if they follow some organized protocol. One of the most effective methods for soft-tissue assessment is a system which can easily be remembered by the acronym HOPS. This stands for *History, Observation, Palpation,* and *Special tests.* We will go through each of these sections and describe how to acquire information for an accurate assessment and then how to interpret that information.

HISTORY:

Taking a proper history is crucial in determining the nature of soft tissue injuries. The history should be much more thorough than a standard set of questions about indications and contraindications. The questions that you will ask in your history will vary with each individual and will vary based on the response that you get to previous questions. Some very important factors such as lifestyle and personality will become evident through a well-taken history.

The information gleaned from the history will have a significant bearing on how the treatment will progress. For example- is this person highly motivated to become well, or are they planning for you to "fix" them. Items such as sleep habits, workload, stress, recreational pursuits, and how this condition is interfering with their life are very important. Information from some of these questions may become some of the best measures of how they have improved following treatment. In certain circumstances, an accurate and thorough history will provide you with the majority of the information you need to proceed in your treatment. While this is obviously not a comprehensive list of questions to be used, some good questions and pertinent information to be gained from a history are included below.

WHAT IS THE NATURE OF YOUR PROBLEM?

It is very beneficial to get information in the client's own words about what is the primary complaint. There is without a doubt an art to listening and picking out the most important aspects of a client's description of the problem. You must learn to hear what aspects of their description are pertinent details and which may not be as important. However, remember that some people will love to talk and they will not be shy about taking up your entire appointment time talking to you. You may be the first health care practitioner who has actually *listened* to them. Also probe here to get information about any accessory problems. For example- neck and back pain may be secondary to a knee injury. The knee injury caused significant changes in gait, which threw off the mechanical and muscular balance in the neck and back causing this secondary pain condition.

WHERE DO YOU FEEL THE PAIN, EXACTLY?

It is important to get as specific information about the location of the pain. It is not good enough to find out that their shoulder hurts. You also must know what part of the shoulder- front or back, topside, etc. Is that pain in a small localized area or does it spread over a larger area. This will be important information in determining which tissues have been injured. For instance, a small localized pain would be more likely to indicate a condition with mechanical disruption of soft-tissue, where a larger area of diffuse pain would be more likely to indicate neurological involvement such as trigger points. If possible, have the client tell you if they can put a finger on the pain. Sometimes a person's description of where the pain is will be less accurate than their ability to exactly localize it with a finger. This will also help to determine if the pain is in a smaller localized area.

HOW DID THE PAIN ARISE?

With this question you will get valuable information about the onset of the pain. You will be treating sudden onset (acute) and gradual onset (chronic) conditions quite differently. Try to get the client to describe the onset of the pain as accurately as possible. If it is a sudden onset condition the more information you can get about the (accident) the better you can determine the tissues which are likely to be at fault. For example- if the person was in a car accident and says their neck hurts, find out in which direction the impact occurred. Was it in front, behind, the side, etc. The direction of impact will put primary stress on different tissues. If the condition was of gradual onset, try to gain information about the types of activities that aggravate the pain most. Occupational or daily activities which cause that pain to be worse are especially relevant.

HOW LONG HAVE YOU HAD THIS PROBLEM?

You want to know if this problem is in an acute stage or if it has been present for a while. This may also give you clues as to the personality and motivation of the client. If a client reports that they have had this condition for a very long time but they are just now getting around to doing something about it, this does not indicate a client with a high level of motivation to get better. Or worse, they may be expecting you to *make* them better. You will probably find less success in treatment with clients who are not motivated to get better. Clients will often describe, when speaking of how long they have had a problem, who else they have seen for the problem.. This information will be quite helpful in determining what approaches you might try with your treatment. If something has already been tried with little or no beneficial results, then you won't have to spend time trying that approach.

WHAT IS THE NATURE OF THE PAIN?   HOW WOULD YOU DESCRIBE IT?   IS IT SHARP, DULL, BURNING, ACHING, DIFFUSE, ELECTRICAL, ETC.?

The nature of the pain will often tell you a great deal about the primary tissues that are injured. For example, pain from a nerve injury is often sharp and shooting. Pain from trigger points is often dull and diffuse. Try to give your client some adjectives to choose from when describing the pain but be careful not to lead them too much or put words in their mouth. For example, "Is the pain sharp?" is not likely to gain as much information as: "If you could use a word to accurately describe the pain you feel would you say it is sharp, dull, burning, aching, stabbing, shooting, etc.?" A more open ended question will often yield more valuable information. It is important to remember that one person's description of sharp is what another person would call shooting. So these adjectives are not completely reliable as descriptions of the pain. They need to be matched and cross-referenced with other information and symptoms that the client reports.

ARE THERE ANY SPECIFIC ACTIVITIES WHICH AGGRAVATE THE PAIN OR DISCOMFORT?   HAVE YOU FOUND ANYTHING THAT MAKES IT FEEL BETTER?

If there is a problem with the musculoskeletal structures, it is likely that there will be more aggravation with activity and relief of the pain with rest. A possible exception to this is pain from an intervertebral disk problem which often will be aggravated by sitting and relieved with movement. Information can be gained from knowing about movement patterns that cause discomfort. This is especially true when you are investigating chronic pain conditions. The information about the specific activities which cause discomfort will help determine which tissues are primarily involved. Without a good understanding of functional anatomy, it becomes difficult to make sense of the information that you are getting from these questions.

WHAT IS THE CLIENT'S OCCUPATION OR DAILY ACTIVITY?

Most individuals consider their occupation to be those activities which they do during the week in order to generate an income. However, occupation should really be expanded to include everything you do to occupy your time. Many different work and recreational activities may be contributing to the current condition. Find out what kinds of stresses the person is exposed to on a regular daily basis.

HAVE YOU EVER HAD THIS OR A SIMILAR CONDITION BEFORE? IF SO, HOW WAS IT RESOLVED?

Comparisons between the current problem and previous ones may give clues as to what is the nature of the injury. It will be helpful to know what types of methods afforded relief the previous time, and if you should suggest adjunctive approaches. You will also get some helpful information here on predisposing factors. Predisposing factors are those elements that make this particular injury more likely to occur or more likely to reoccur in the future.

OBSERVATION:

The massage practitioner may learn a great deal simply by visual examination. Patterns of body symmetry may reveal important information about muscular tension or tissue dysfunction. Previous injuries may have left important clues as to the nature of the present condition. Although you may not have equipment readily available to you, it will help to be able to perform some of your observation methods in a graphical reference format. A graphical reference format is a geometric standard such as a plumb line or a grid on the wall behind the client.

It is important not to be overzealous in attempting to have an individual conform to the "ideal" posture which may be outlined in many anatomical or medical texts. There are many unique structural differences between all of us that prevent us from being the ideal postural man or woman. This does not necessarily point to any particular pathology. What is important to recognize is whether a deviation from an established norm is significantly dysfunctional as to be a cause of some type of soft-tissue pathology.

Observation of the client's movement may also yield valuable information about muscular or soft tissue involvement. If the client reports that a certain movement hurts, you may be able to have them do that movement in a series of different movements and watch for the level of apprehension or ability to perform the specific movement.

It is a good idea to begin your clinical observation of the client the moment you see them. If they are aware that you are specifically "observing" them, they are more likely to be aware of how they move and subsequently move less naturally. You may also be able to get some preliminary sense of muscle tone simply by noting its appearance. Take note of the postural factors in the observation section and see how they relate to the information you will gain from other areas.

When performing the observation portion of the assessment, it is important to keep an open mind about the variety of factors which may be involved in creating a certain postural distortion. Some practitioners may be too quick to jump to conclusions based on one particular model about soft-tissue dysfunction. If the predominant model in that person's practice is one that revolves around the role of psychological issues in creating somatic dysfunction, then it is likely that the practitioner will see a client with rounded, forward slumping shoulders as someone who is "holding on to fear" for example. If the practitioner's predominant model or paradigm revolves around a purely structural component he or she may see this same client as someone who has a chronic shortening of the pectoralis minor and medial rotators of the shoulder. Both approaches may have a certain degree of validity. In fact, it is often very difficult to know exactly what is going on until you have spent significant time with the client over the course of several treatment sessions. Many conditions will involve components of structural and emotionally created elements of the dysfunction.

PALPATION:

If you are a massage practitioner, then palpation is your specialty. Massage therapists spend more time doing palpation than virtually anyone else in the health care system. Because of that, they should be very good at it. We can do a great deal more to improve our palpation skills. Remember that as a massage practitioner you have your diagnostic and treatment tool right there in your hands. The human hand is an incredibly sensitive tool. Its ability to define and discern various tissue textures, levels of edema, subcutaneous fibrosity, etc. makes it highly specialized. The fact that you can immediately take the information in from your hands, process it through the brain, integrate those sensations with your knowledge and intuition, and then immediately make adjustments in your treatment with that same hand is really quite remarkable.

You will be performing palpation not only in assessment before the treatment, but during the entire treatment as well. Keep attentive to subtle sensations that you feel in the tissues at all times. This will be valuable information that you will want to record. Make notes of any areas that are tender either locally or with referral. You will use information gained during palpation to verify the location of injured tissues or pain referral patterns.

SPECIAL ORTHOPEDIC TESTS:

Some authors do not include the active range of motion, passive range of motion, or manual resistive tests in the "S" section of the HOPS acronym. They will list them separately. However in this text they are included for two reasons. They fit in well with the model of what the special tests are designed to describe, and it is a convenient way to remember them. The special tests section is composed of 4 different components.

1. Active range of motion tests
2. Passive range of motion tests
3. Manual resistive tests
4. Special regional orthopedic tests.

The order in which they are performed is important as well. As each of the different sections is presented, the rationale for performing them in this order should become clear.

IMPORTANT: Remember that a positive result is not determined by one positive finding. This information must be balanced by findings from other types of evaluation. Assessment procedures are a way of gaining more valuable information to narrow down your focus and try to determine what is going on. It is tempting to want to have the client's problem exactly fit the symptoms of some type of condition that you are familiar with or have had good success with in the past. Avoid this mistake! A common axiom to follow is— "Rule out, don't rule in.." This means, try to rule out things that you don't think are going on until you arrive at a satisfactory explanation. Don't try to make the client's symptoms fit your picture of what you would like their problem to be.

---

1. ACTIVE RANGE OF MOTION TESTS

Active movements focus on the contractile tissues, the muscle-tendon unit, which are necessary for movement. These tissues are considered one contiguous unit because they work in conjunction with each other. Several different types of information can be gained from active movement including willingness to move, range of motion, muscle strength, and coordination.

A client's willingness to move could be limited by actual pain or it may be a motivational problem. There are some clients who associate effort with pain or discomfort so when asked to perform an active movement they may indicate that it is painful or uncomfortable. Try to determine if this is genuine pain or if this is psychological resistance to movement. Information on available range of motion will become evident with active movements. This will later be confirmed with the passive range of motion tests. Muscle strength and coordination of movement are often visible through active movements. Greater information about muscle strength will then be compared with findings from manual resistive tests.

It is important to remember that both contractile and inert tissues will be moving with active movements. All tissues that are attached to the rigid moving links of the skeletal system will have some form of movement response during active motions. Contractile tissues may have stress placed on them by contraction or stretching during active movements.

IMPORTANT POINTS TO WATCH FOR:

1. When and where during movement the onset of pain occurs

Information gained here will help clarify if the location of pain is consistent with what should happen with each particular injury condition An example is abduction of the shoulder which produces a painful arc. This is likely to be indicative of some type of tissue (often the sub-acromial bursa) being pinched or squeezed. A painful arc would not likely be present if the pain or discomfort was only in the muscle tendon unit. The most common injury to a ligament is an excessive tensile stress injury. Adequate knowledge of functional anatomy will help determine which tissue is injured. If you are aware of what muscles do what actions, then you can more easily distinguish what parts of particular movements are likely to be dysfunctional. For example, certain muscles may be more active in the beginning of a range of motion than throughout the middle or end of that particular range.

2. Whether movement increases the intensity and quality of pain

If movement increases the intensity or quality of the pain it is much more likely that you have some type of lesion to the moving soft tissue structures. This will be an important factor in ruling out certain neurological pain problems. If you have a nerve root being compressed by a protruding intervertebral disc, there may be significant pain regardless of movement of the affected part. You will want to verify and cross reference this information with the passive range of motion tests you will perform.

3. The client's reaction to pain

If the client is performing some type of active range of motion test and encounters pain during the test, you want to make note of the quality of the pain. Does it seem to be severe and limiting, or is it just a mild discomfort? Is the pain consistent with repeated movements? There are some clients who will exaggerate the level of pain they report in order to gain sympathy, or for financial gain. This is common with some workmen's compensation claims if a person does not want to return to work and is essentially getting paid for being injured.

4. Amount of observable restriction

This is an example of the importance of the observation portion of the assessment that will be performed while you are doing some other type of test. By having the client attempt certain functional movements of their daily life (often called ADL's—activities of daily living), such as combing their hair or looking over their shoulder as if backing up in a car, you can determine more about how their particular condition is actually affecting them.

5. Pattern of movement

When observing the active range of motion, determine if the movement seems smooth and within the normal range for that particular movement, or are they substituting or compensating for injured tissues. An example would be active shoulder abduction for a client that has adhesive capsulitis (frozen shoulder). They will show a dysfunctional movement between the scapula and the humerus which makes it appear that they can reach 90^0 of abduction when that is not actually happening. What is happening instead is that they will often laterally flex the torso or elevate the scapula to help produce what appears to be an abduction movement.

6. Muscular splinting or guarding that is present

A sure sign of soft-tissue distress is the splinting or compensating spasm of surrounding muscles. If there is an obvious sign of splinting or muscular guarding, you can be relatively certain that smooth mechanical function has been impaired. Management of this condition should not only focus on the injury site, but also on decreasing the secondary muscular splinting which has occurred.

7. Movement of associated joints

During active movements you want to be aware of the possibility of joint pathology. Since active movements include movement at the joint, the primary pathology may be there and not in the moving soft tissues. This will be elaborated upon and confirmed later through the use of certain passive movements.

8. Nature of movement on uninvolved side

Noticing an awkward or ill-patterned movement on one side is not enough to verify that there is a problem. There are certain factors which may have us adopting unusual movement patterns that are the same on each side. These patterns may not be a pathological condition, simply an unusual pattern of mechanics. One of the primary reasons for testing the uninvolved side first is to establish a baseline of measurement of what type of movement is present in the "healthy" side.

9. Willingness of client to move the injured area

As mentioned earlier, this will be a significant indicator of motivation as well as tissue dysfunction. If someone is extremely apprehensive to move an area it is usually indicative of a very painful condition that they are trying to avoid. This may give you some initial information about how severe the injured area is damaged. It is not always necessary to require someone to make a certain movement in order to verify that there is tissue injury in that region. If the pain of movement is so great as to keep the person from wanting to move at all, that should be considered as a positive indicator of tissue injury.

10. Quality of the movement

When you observe quality of movement you are looking for factors such as smoothness, coordination, and rhythm. Is this movement smooth and steady throughout the range or is it suddenly jerky in certain portions of the range. Lack of smoothness may indicate several factors from muscular imbalance and dysfunction to severe joint pathology such as loose fragments within the joint capsule.

How To Perform Active Range Of Motion Tests

1. Determine the motions possible at that joint

Any examination of normal or pathological motion at a joint must begin with an understanding of normal mechanics of that joint. For example, in order to know that excessive rotation of the knee joint in an extended position is an indicator of an injury, you must know that the knee does not normally make that motion. In each of the regional sections in later chapters, there is a definition of the primary single plane movements that are capable at that joint. A single plane movement is one that happens mostly or exclusively in one plane. For example flexion is a single plane movement that the elbow is capable of in the sagittal plane.

2. Determine which tissues will be involved actively

In an active range of motion test the primary tissues to be involved will be the muscle-tendon unit. However, it must be kept in mind that many of the inert tissues will be moved as a natural consequence of movement at the joint. Make sure that the movement you are requiring will isolate the particular tissues that you want to investigate. For example, if you want to investigate a problem with the supraspinatus muscle, an active range of motion test for medial rotation of the shoulder is not likely to tell you much about the supraspinatus muscle-tendon unit. That does not mean that it will not tell you anything, because this may be valuable to rule out the involvement of certain other tissues. However, the primary tissue you are interested in (supraspinatus in this case) will have virtually no involvement.

3. Demonstrate the movement that will be performed

Demonstrating the movement first will make sure that the client fully understands what you are asking them to do. That way the end range of motion that you are looking for, the exact pattern of movement you want to see, and how much effort should be expended are well illustrated. This will be helpful for clients who are more visually oriented. For example, it is hard to tell a client to bring their arm up by flexing the arm at the shoulder until they are in full flexion. They are not as likely to understand this instruction even if you simplify it to say raise your arm straight up in front of you until it is straight up. It is much easier to demonstrate the movement.

4. Test the uninvolved side first

There are several reasons for this. It helps to demonstrate the movement that you are going to do and it decreases any apprehension that the client may have about what is going to be expected of them. It will also give you a baseline against which to measure the dysfunction on the problem side. By establishing what is normal for that client, you can then determine what is abnormal or dysfunctional. The level of proprioceptive awareness that the client has will also be increased by paying attention to what happens on the normal side.

5. Test the involved side

Once the baseline has been established and you are clear what you are looking for, then test the involved side. If there are movements that you suspect are going to be painful, it may be helpful to do them last. If movements cause pain, the client is likely to be apprehensive about performing these movements. This may limit your ability to get them to fully cooperate with future movements. In addition, certain movements which irritate problem tissues may increase inflammation when the client performs them repeatedly. For that reason, it is best to do these at the end of your section of active movements that you are testing.

6. Ask and make note of any reported pain or discomfort

Throughout the time you are performing each of these procedures you should be getting clear information about whether any of these motions caused any pain or discomfort. When the client reports that they did cause pain or discomfort, try to gain information about what kind of pain or discomfort they felt, its duration, intensity, etc. It will be very helpful to keep notes of these statements so you can have this information for your records later as you try to sort out your findings.

2. PASSIVE RANGE OF MOTION TESTS

Passive motions focus on the inert tissues. In passive movements the contractile tissues are also moved, but not engaged. This is an important distinction. Remember that certain contractile tissues or portions of them can be stressed (tensile stress) by stretching. This will naturally happen during passive movements. Where your client is reporting the pain will be a significant indicator to help you discover the primary problem area. Much of the information about range of motion can be determined through active range of motion tests, making some passive range of motion tests unnecessary. You will want to coordinate findings in your passive range of motion tests with those of the active range of motion tests.

One of the more valuable types of information that will be gained through the use of passive range of motion tests is the quality of movement at a joint. Information about certain joint dysfunctions can be gained from passive range of motion tests. The practitioner will be interested in both normal motion and what is called accessory motion. Accessory motion is motion at the end range of movement that is not created through the client's active movement, but is still within normal anatomical limits. For example, when a client actively hyperextends the wrist, a certain range of motion is achieved. By applying a degree of pressure to the palm of the hand in the direction of further hyperextension the practitioner can get a slightly greater range of motion without going past the natural anatomical boundary. This is accessory joint motion.

The quality of the end of accessory motion is an important indicator of joint or soft-tissue pathology. This information can be categorized by what is called the "end-feel". The end-feel describes a certain quality of movement at the end of that joint's range of motion. Several different end-feels are described below. It is important to remember that whether or not an end-feel is pathological or normal depends on a number of factors, most important of which is what joint is being examined. For example, the end-feel described below as a bone-to bone end-feel is normal for elbow extension. However it is pathological if it is felt at the end of lateral rotation of the shoulder. Again, familiarity with anatomical structures will be very important in order to determine what is an appropriate end-feel at each individual joint.

1) *Bone to bone*-- This is the end-feel that results from two bony surfaces contacting each other at their normal end range of movement. An example would be full extension of the elbow where the olecranon process contacts the olecranon fossa.   *NORMAL*

2) *Soft tissue approximation*-- At certain joints the range of motion is slowed or stopped by the compression of muscle tissue of the muscles acting on the joint. An example is full flexion of the elbow where the biceps brachii and the forearm flexors pressing on each other limits any further movement. This will also be seen in the hamstrings with full knee flexion in an individual who has very good flexibility of the quadriceps. The hamstrings and the calf muscles pressing on each other will be what limit the movement.   *NORMAL*

3) *Tissue stretch*-- This is perhaps the most common normal end-feel and is the result of a stretch of the soft-tissue structures surrounding the joint. This end-feel may feel somewhat "leathery" as the stretch of the soft-tissue limits the movement. Lateral rotation of the shoulder which stretches the medial rotator muscles and the anterior joint capsule is a good example of this type of end-feel.   *NORMAL - MOST COME*

4) *Muscle spasm*-- Limitation to movement that happens as a result of muscular spasm will be felt as abrupt and premature to where the end range of motion should be. There will usually be pain associated with the end range here also. Muscle spasm is considered a true pathological end-feel in that there is no joint that should have muscle spasm as its normal end-feel.   *PATHOLOGIC*

5) *Springy block*-- This is a pathological end-feel that is associated with a loose body in the joint. An example where this is likely to occur is during motions of the knee where a torn meniscus is present and there is a loose body of cartilage in the joint. The loose body will wedge in between the tibia and   *PATHOLOGIC*

femur and prevent normal joint mechanics from occurring at the knee joint. An analogy which can be use here is the type of movement that occurs to a door when something is jammed in the door frame near the hinge, preventing it from closing. It has a tendency to "spring back". This is the nature of the springy block end-feel.

6) Empty-- In this end-feel there is no apparent mechanical obstruction to movement but the client suddenly halts or stops movement because of pain that is produced by the movement. Conditions such as bursitis will often produce this type of end feel. *PATHOLOGIC*

How To Perform Passive Range Of Motion Tests

1. Determine the motions possible at that joint

This is the same as for active range of motion tests. Any examination of normal or pathological motion at a joint must begin with an understanding of normal mechanics of that joint. Refer to the single plane movements of each joint in the regional sections in order to determine the normal end-feel for that particular joint motion.

2. Determine which tissues will be involved passively

Remember that passive movements focus on the inert tissues. However, contractile tissues such as muscles and tendons will be stretched at the end range of passive movements. It will likely be ligaments which will be most involved in limiting the end range of motion in many of the primary single plane movements.

3. Demonstrate the movement that will be performed

Demonstrating the movement first will make sure that the client fully understands what you are asking them to do. That way the end range of motion that you are looking for, the exact pattern of movement you want to see, and how much effort should be expended are well illustrated. This will be helpful for clients who are more visually oriented.

4. Get the client to relax as much as possible

It is especially important to have the client relax during passive range of motion tests. You are trying to identify subtle sensations of joint motion and distinguish between pure joint movement and joint movement which incorporates contractile tissues. Therefore try to get the client to relax fully so that only joint motion is tested and not muscular involvement with any of the motions.

5. Test the uninvolved side first

The rationale for testing the uninvolved side first is the same for passive movements as it is for active movements.

6. Test the involved side

Once the baseline has been established and you are clear what you are looking for, then test the involved side. If there are movements that you suspect are going to be painful, it may be helpful to do them last. If movements cause pain, the client is likely to be apprehensive about performing these movements. This may limit your ability to get them to fully cooperate with future movements. In addition, certain movements which irritate problem tissues may increase inflammation when the client performs them repeatedly. For that reason, it is best to do these at the end of your section of passive movements that you are testing. Remember that during passive range of motion tests you are particularly interested in the nature of the end-feel at the joint.

7. Ask and make any note of any reported pain or discomfort
This is the same as noted above in active range of motion tests.

---

3. MANUAL RESISTIVE TESTS

Manual resistive tests are frequently called resisted isometric movements since they use isometric muscle contractions. However, this is somewhat confusing because an isometric contraction does not produce any movement at the joint. These tests will be called manual resistive tests because the practitioner uses his/her hands to provide resistance to movement thereby causing an isometric muscle contraction.

This test is designed to confirm and elaborate on findings from the active and passive range of motion tests. The emphasis is on determining if problems are primarily associated with a certain muscle tendon unit. This is done by selectively applying tension to that particular unit. Because an isometric muscle contraction is used, there is no movement occurring at the joint. For that reason the inert tissues are not involved. However it is important to remember that problems in inert tissues could show up from a manual resistive test. An example is fibrous adhesion between a muscle and an underlying joint capsule or ligamentous structure. Pain would be elicited from the muscle contraction pulling on the areas of adhesion although the problem itself was not actually in the muscle tissue.

What A Manual Resistive Test Tells You:

As with the other tests above, it is important to remember that these are not definitive tests. Meaning you will not be able to say this is exactly what is wrong simply because you got a positive or negative result with this particular test. These tests are used to help clarify information gained from other areas and lead you to where you might go next in verifying your suspicions. Some guidelines are given below for results which you are likely to see from manual resistive tests.

1. Resisted movements which are strong, equal to the unaffected side, and pain free indicate that the problem does not lie in the muscle tendon unit.

2. If a resisted movement is strong or relatively strong and causes pain, this indicates some type of injury to the muscle tendon unit. This will often be a muscle strain. Problems of neuromuscular activity which induce chronic muscle spasm may also produce pain. It is important not to immediately assume that a strain is the cause of the pain. Coordinate this information with the history in order to make a good determination.

3. Resisted movements that are weak and painful will often be a result of problems with a neuromuscular component or severe joint injury which causes a reflex muscular inhibition.

4. Resisted movements which are weak and painless will often be indicators of a severe neurological lesion or a ruptured tendon.

How To Perform Manual Resistive Tests:

1. Determine the location of the muscle to be tested

In performing manual resistive tests it will be important to know the location (including attachment sites) for the muscle that you are going to be testing. A problem could be present anywhere along the muscle's length, the musculotendinous junction, or the tendo-periosteal junction. Your anatomical knowledge about the location of that muscle's fibers will help you design the most appropriate manual resistive test.

2. Determine the primary action of the muscle to be tested

When performing manual resistive tests, it is imperative that the practitioner be able to isolate the muscle in question by specific action. If not, the test will not yield information that will help the process, it will only add confusion to the assessment. Again, knowledge of functional anatomy and kinesiology is imperative to perform manual resistive tests with any accuracy. There is a great art to manual muscle testing. It is often discredited as being unreliable because of the subjective experience of the practitioner who is applying the test. However, no suitable muscle testing procedure has been developed which can match the sensitivity of a trained practitioner and provide the same types of options for isolating movement. In the quest of becoming more objective the hard sciences have attempted to take the examiner out of the equation. While this approach is valid to a degree, when it comes to muscle testing, a trained practitioner may be preferable because of the multiple levels of information that can be processed. For example, the practitioner performing a manual muscle test can be feeling not only for the quality of movement but the sense of effort exerted by the client, expressions of pain or discomfort on their face, and sensing whether they are giving a genuine effort or not.

3. Find a position which will effectively isolate that muscle

A manual resistive test is designed to isolate one particular muscle, group of muscles, or one particular action. If you are trying to determine the effectiveness of the infraspinatus in performing lateral rotation of the shoulder it is not sufficient just to have the client attempt to laterally rotate the shoulder while you offer resistance. You must position yourself in a place that allows you to offer that resistance while still being able to sense fine discriminations of effort on their part. If your body position requires you to expend too much effort to resist their attempted movement, you will not be able to gain the proper amount of information from the test.

4. Test the uninvolved side first

The same principles apply here as with the active and passive range of motion tests regarding the testing of the uninvolved side first: reducing client apprehension, demonstrating the correct movement to be performed, and establishing an effective baseline against which to measure results from the involved side.

5. Test the involved side

There are two effective ways to offer resistance during a manual resistive test. During either method it is best to find a place that is about midway through the range of motion. That is the point at which you want to offer resistance.

A) Find a way to offer resistance to the desired motion and have the client attempt to move in that direction. About 25% of full strength is usually sufficient to determine problems. However, it is often hard for some people to judge 25% of their full effort. For example, if you wish to test for lateral rotation of the shoulder, you would ask the client to laterally rotate the shoulder and you would apply resistance to the limb that would prevent that movement. The client is not likely to know what lateral rotation of the shoulder is so it will be helpful to give them a kinesthetic cue. For example, you might say "Susan I want you to turn your arm out in this way (you show her what motion you want her to perform) using only a moderate amount of effort".

B) It is sometimes easier and more effective if the therapist initiates a movement in the opposite direction and has the client attempt to hold the position. This is particularly effective because it is the therapist who gets to determine how much force is used and if the direction of movement is exactly what you wish to isolate. Using our example of lateral rotation of the shoulder above, in this case we would ask the client to hold the shoulder still while the therapist attempted to medially rotate the shoulder. This attempt to hold the static position will engage the lateral rotators of the shoulder.

6. Ask and make note of any reported pain or discomfort

4. SPECIAL REGIONAL ORTHOPEDIC TESTS

This is a group of tests that are designed to discover a particular problem in an isolated area such as the likelihood of carpal tunnel syndrome at the wrist or an injured medial collateral ligament at the knee. These tests will take into account specific factors of functional anatomy of the region. Some sort of specific stress or change in state will be administered to a certain area with the likelihood of either a positive test, indicating the likelihood of a certain condition, or a negative test indicating the likelihood that a particular condition is not there. Remember this is not a definitive test, it only indicates a high likelihood that a condition is present. Special regional orthopedic tests for individual conditions will be presented during the regional chapters which cover specific disorders.

ADDITIONAL DIAGNOSTIC TESTS AND PROCEDURES

Although it is not within the scope of practice of massage to order or perform any of the following tests, they were included for reference purposes. Many massage practitioners will have clients come to see them who have had these procedures performed. In addition, massage practitioners may find themselves working with other health care professionals who will be performing these procedures and it will be very helpful to understand what types of information can be gained from these tests.

X-RAY- This test may also be called roentgenogram. This is one of the most common orthopedic evaluation tools. X-Ray uses a high energy electromagnetic wave which penetrates the tissues and can be detected through the use of a special photographic plate behind the tissues. Different tissues will absorb different amounts of the electromagnetic wave. Selective absorption is what causes the variety of shadowy images which are characteristic of X-Rays. Disorders of the bones or joint pathology such as the formation of osteophytes are picked up very well through X-Ray. Certain tissues such as muscles are hardly visible on X-Ray so disorders such as muscle strain, or trigger points will not appear on these types of tests.

BONE SCAN- Chemical compounds or radioactive isotopes may be injected into the body and then viewed by special sensing equipment. Certain organs or very minor bony injuries such as stress fractures may take up a large amount of the chemical compound. When the bone scan is viewed this exaggerated amount of activity will be detected indicating the presence of a particular pathology. Since stress fractures often do not show up on an X-Ray, the bone scan is often the best method of identifying them.

CAT SCAN- CAT stands for computer assisted tomography. This test is somewhat akin to an X-Ray but the images that are produced can be enhanced with the help of a computer. That is why it is called computer assisted tomography. They are effective in outlining complicated fractures or structures deep within the body.

MRI- MRI stands for Magnetic Resonance Imaging. This technique is considered non-invasive and painless because nothing (physical) actually penetrates the skin. However if you ask someone who has had an MRI if it was painless and non-invasive they may not agree. Patients receiving an MRI often have to lay very still for very long periods (close to an hour) while a machine produces an image of the interior of the body based on the reception from magnetic fields detected by the testing device. Many patients report that the machine produces a very claustrophobic sensation during the test. The benefit of an MRI is that it can often produce very dramatic and detailed pictures of the interior of the body. However, it is an extremely expensive test.

EMG- An EMG study is one that uses electromyography. This is the graphical measurement of the contraction of a muscle as a result of an electrical stimulation. EMG studies are often beneficial in examining problems of the neuromuscular component of soft-tissues. If someone has carpal tunnel syndrome and the flow of nerve impulses is being impeded in the median nerve because of its compression in the carpal tunnel, this might show up on an EMG test.

MYELOGRAM- A myelogram is a special type of X-Ray examination taken of the spinal region after a certain dye or other contrast medium has been injected into the spinal column. This enables the examiner to detect the presence of disc protrusions or lesions.

ISOKINETIC EVALUATION- This test uses a computer assisted strength resistance device which offers accommodating resistance. Accommodating resistance means that the machine can sense how much effort a muscle is exerting through its range of motion as it moves at a constant velocity. A great deal of information can be gained and quantified from the use of isokinetic testing procedures regarding the improvement in muscle strength and joint function following injuries and surgery.

ARTHROGRAM- The arthrogram is another special type of X-Ray procedure. A radiopaque contrast medium or air is injected into the joint region. Tendon, ligament, or meniscal tears will often become apparent with this procedure.

Section 2
Conditions and Assessment
by Anatomical Region

Section 2 begins the chapters dealing with the various regions of the body. Each chapter will be organized in a fashion that follows the principles presented in the first three chapters on the theory of assessment. The format followed in these chapters is as follows:

Special Terms and Concepts - This section will define terms that are used in the chapter that refer to anatomy, mechanics, or rehabilitation of that region.

Overview of Common Single Plane Movements - Each of the primary single plane movements that are possible at the joints of that body region will be described.

Active Range of Motion Tests - It is assumed that active range of motion tests for a joint region will include all the single plane movements that are possible at the joint. This section will include any special information that is unique or relevant to that region when performing active range of motion tests.

Passive Range of Motion Tests - As with active range of motion tests, all single plane movements at each particular joint will be included in a passive range of motion test. Any special aspects of passive range of motion tests for that regional area will be included in this section. Also included in this section will be a description of the end-feel for each of the single plane movements of the joints in that region.

Manual Resistive Tests - Any special points relevant to manual resistive tests performed at the joints of each region will be included here. Pictures and descriptions of how to perform manual resistive tests will be included in this section.

Guide to Conditions and Special Orthopedic Tests of Each Region - This section will be divided up into two parts. The first part will cover structural and postural deviations, and the second part will cover common injury conditions. Each of the conditions described has a number which is used for quick reference in the chart at the end of the chapter. The conditions will be described and illustrated, assessment procedures will be discussed, and suggestions for treatment will be offered.

Reference Chart - At the end of each chapter on the different regional areas there is a quick reference chart. The chart describes the region of pain the client is likely to experience, whether its onset is acute or chronic, what is a possible cause, and a reference number to a description of that condition. Note that some references may be for conditions that are in other chapters.

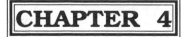

CHAPTER 4

FOOT, ANKLE AND LEG CONDITIONS

SPECIAL TERMS AND CONCEPTS

1) LONGITUDINAL ARCH- is formed by the structure of the bones of the foot and is supported by the tension in the plantar fascia. This is a structural arch of the foot that runs from the calcaneus to the heads of the metatarsals. It is actually somewhat triangular in shape with the narrow point of the triangle at the calcaneus and the two long sides of the triangle spreading out to the 1st and 5th metatarsal heads. A line connecting the 1st and 5th metatarsal heads completes the triangle. The arch is primarily designed to aid the foot in shock absorbency and in adapting the foot to variations in ground structure (this last feature is less relevant when walking in shoes). When someone is said to have a "high arch" or "fallen arches" it is most often the longitudinal arch that they are speaking of.

2) TRANSVERSE ARCH- is functionally like the longitudinal arch in that it is designed to absorb shock and help the foot adapt to variations in ground surface. This arch travels across the foot in a medial to lateral direction (frontal plane). It is much shorter than the longitudinal arch and higher on the medial side of the foot.

3) ORTHOTICS- are inserts which are placed in the shoe in order to help redistribute biomechanical stresses on the foot. They may be made of several different materials including rigid plastics or soft foam based materials. They can be purchased over the counter or specially designed for each individual's foot by the use of a plaster cast that determines the contours of the foot.

4) PRONATION- is a term used with great frequency and with a variety of meanings. It is primarily used in describing the position of the hand and wrist, but is frequently used to determine the position of the foot. In this text, the term is used as it is currently employed in other sports medicine and orthopedic texts as a dynamic movement of the foot. That means it does not represent a static position, but rather a combination of movements that happen during the normal gait pattern of the foot. Pronation refers to the combination of movements of dorsiflexion, eversion, and abduction of the foot. Dorsiflexion and eversion will be clarified further in the overview of single plane movements. Abduction of the foot is a rotary movement that happens in the transverse plane and is intimately tied to small amounts of rotary movement at the knee. Abduction of the foot can be demonstrated by having a client sit on the edge of the treatment table and let the leg hang off with the knee flexed at approximately 90°. With the plantar surface of the foot remaining parallel to the floor, have the client point their toes alternately to the right and left. When the foot moves in a lateral direction, that is abduction. When it moves in a medial direction, that is adduction. If a person is said to "overpronate" that means that they move through the natural sequence of pronation either too fast or too far.

5) SUPINATION- is the opposite of pronation. It is a dynamic movement of the foot which is composed of three different positions or movements of the foot during the normal walking or running gait. Supination is composed of plantar flexion, inversion, and adduction. Plantar flexion and inversion are defined in the following section on single plane movements of the foot and ankle. See the above description of pronation for a definition of adduction of the foot.

Overview of Common Single Plane Movements of the Foot, Ankle, & Leg

Active and passive ROM tests and manual resistive tests will require a knowledge of basic joint mechanics and functional anatomy for the regions surrounding the joint. The practitioner must know what constitutes normal, pain free motion at a joint in order to determine if there is a problem with that joint. The discussions of active ROM tests, passive ROM tests, and manual resistive tests will utilize the terms listed below. Familiarity with these terms and how they apply to the body will be essential in order to gain valid information from the assessment. All joint angle measurements which are included are measured from the neutral position, which is anatomical position. In order to properly understand and simplify joint mechanics, the movements at the joints described in each regional section in the book have been broken down into single plane movements. That means movement in one of the three primary planes of motion - sagittal, frontal, or transverse. Although this greatly simplifies the analysis of movement, it should be kept in mind that this classification rarely happens in actual human movement. Almost every movement we make will be a combination of movements in different planes. However, muscle or joint dysfunction can often be accurately pinpointed by comparing certain single plane movements. The primary muscles involved with each action are listed under the description of that action. Note that this may not include every muscle which is involved in that action, but only the primary ones.

Dorsiflexion- is a movement where the top side of the foot comes toward the anterior portion of the lower leg. (The toes are brought back toward the knees.) Average range of motion in dorsiflexion is from 20° to 30°. The primary muscles involved with dorsiflexion are:

> **Tibialis Anterior**
> **Extensor Digitorum Longus**
> **Extensor Hallucis Longus**

Plantar flexion- is a movement in which the top side of the foot moves away from the anterior portion of the lower leg. This happens when you point your toes. Some authors will call this movement extension, which is actually more correct, since flexion is used to denote a decrease in the joint angle. Average range of motion in plantar flexion is 30° to 50°. The primary muscles involved in plantar flexion are:

> **Gastrocnemius**
> **Soleus**
> **Plantaris**
> **Flexor Digitorum Longus**
> **Peroneus Longus**
> **Peroneus Brevis**
> **Flexor Hallucis Longus**
> **Tibialis Posterior**

Inversion- is when the plantar surface of the foot is brought toward the midline of the body. Some authors will describe this movement as supination. See the above descriptions of supination and pronation for a distinction. Average range of motion for inversion is 50°. The primary muscles involved with inversion are:

> **Tibialis Posterior**
> **Flexor Digitorum Longus**
> **Flexor Hallucis Longus**
> **Tibialis Anterior**
> **Extensor Hallucis Longus**

Eversion- is when the plantar surface of the foot is brought away from the midline of the body. Some authors describe this movement as pronation. See the above descriptions of supination and pronation for a distinction. Average range of motion for eversion is 25°. The primary muscles involved in eversion are:

> **Peroneus Longus**
> **Peroneus Brevis**
> **Peroneus Tertius**
> **Extensor Digitorum Longus**

Active Range of Motion Tests

Active ROM tests for the foot and ankle will include dorsiflexion, plantar flexion, inversion, and eversion. The movements described in the **Special Terms and Concepts** section as abduction and adduction are not included because they only occur under special circumstances. Check the list of muscles involved with the 4 primary movements of the foot in order to determine which muscles will be involved in each of the individual movements. Notice that their may be a difference in weight-bearing versus non-weight bearing discomfort as some of these tests are performed. For example if you have the client attempt to plantar flex the foot while lying on the treatment table, you may get a very different response than if you have him/her attempt to stand up on tiptoes from a neutral standing position. Weight bearing relationships should always be taken into account when examining movements of the foot and ankle.

Passive Range of Motion Tests

The practitioner should pay particular attention to the nature of end-feels generated with passive range of motion tests when comparing these findings with active range of motion tests.

The end-feel for dorsiflexion will be tissue stretch. Dorsiflexion is limited by the flexibility of the gastrocnemius and soleus muscles as well as the increasing width of the talus as it rolls under the tibia.

The end-feel for plantar flexion will also be tissue stretch. It is limited primarily by the lengthening of the tibialis anterior, extensor digitorum longus, extensor hallucis longus, and the ligamentous webbing of the ankle joint.

The end-feel for inversion will also be tissue stretch. It is primarily limited by tightening of the anterior talofibular ligament. Note that the tissue stretch end-feel for ligaments is more abrupt than that for muscle and tendons because of the capability of the muscle tendon unit to elongate significantly.

The end-feel for eversion will be more like a bone to bone end-feel. Although there is a tightening of the deltoid ligament to prevent excessive eversion, the end of movement is also created by the talus contacting the lateral malleolus. The fibula extends farther on the lateral side than the tibia does on the medial side and this causes eversion to have a shorter range of motion and a bone to bone end-feel.

Manual Resistive Tests

In this next section manual resistive tests will be demonstrated for the four primary single plane movements of the foot and ankle: dorsiflexion, plantar flexion, inversion, and eversion. It should be remembered that there are many different positions for manual resistive tests. The methods which are illustrated are given as suggestions. Also keep in mind that there are two different ways to perform manual resistive tests which were described in the section on assessment theory. Regardless of which method of performing the test is used, the direction of pull by the client and the direction of resistance by the therapist are the same.

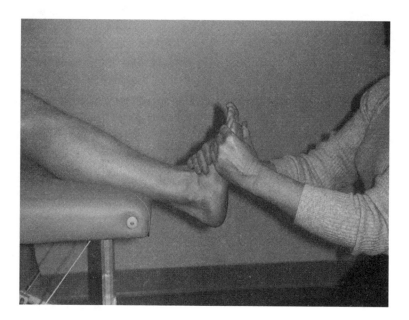

Figure 4-1
*Resisted dorsiflexion
of the foot*

The client is in a supine position with the foot extended off the end of the treatment table. The therapist is holding the dorsal or top surface of the foot. The foot is put in a mid range of dorsiflexion. The client will attempt to dorsiflex the foot while the therapist offers resistance.

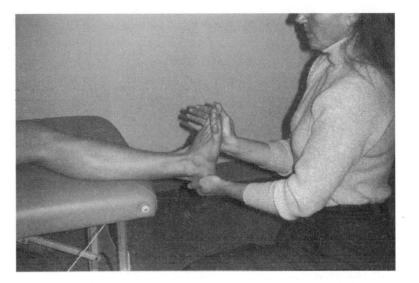

Figure 4-2
*Resisted plantar flexion
of the foot*

The client is in a supine position on the treatment table. The foot may be off the end of the treatment table in order to have a little more freedom of movement. The foot will be placed in a mid range of plantar flexion. The client will attempt to plantar flex the foot and the therapist will offer resistance with a hand placed on the ball of the foot. Most people are unaware of how strong they are in plantar flexion. You may want to remind the client that only a moderate amount of effort is needed.

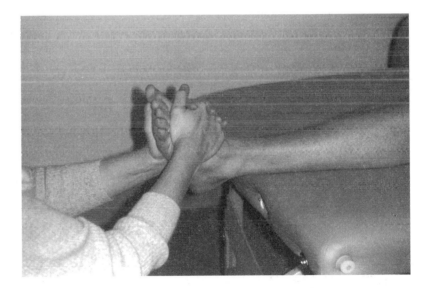

Figure 4-3
*Resisted inversion
of the foot*

The client is supine on the treatment table and the foot is off the end of the table. The therapist will place one hand on the dorsal surface of the foot and one hand on the plantar surface of the foot. The therapist's fingers will be interlocked to form a tight grasp of the foot. This hand position affords a good hold on the foot without interfering in joint mechanics. The client will attempt to invert the foot and the therapist will offer resistance.

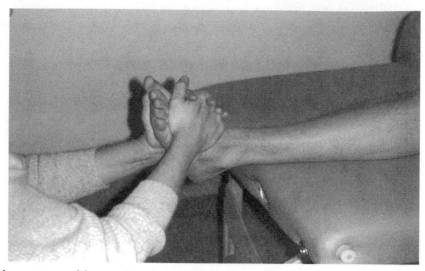

Figure 4-4
*Resisted eversion
of the Foot*

The client and therapist are in the same position as that described for inversion. The only difference is that in this test the client will attempt to evert the foot and the therapist will offer resistance. It is helpful for the therapist to have his/her body close to the hands so the body's center of gravity can help in offering resistance.

GUIDE TO CONDITIONS AND SPECIAL REGIONAL ORTHOPEDIC TESTS OF THE FOOT, ANKLE, AND LEG

Structural and Postural Deviations

(1) CONDITION: CALCANEAL VARUS

CHARACTERISTICS: This is a condition in which the distal portion of the calcaneus is deviating in a medial direction. This angulation of the calcaneus is likely to interfere with the normal foot mechanics and may involve other soft-tissue dysfunctions as well. It is most likely to be present with tightness of the inverter muscle group.

Figure 4-5
This is a posterior view of the left foot showing calcaneal varus. The distal portion of the calcaneus is deviating in a medial direction

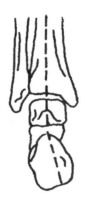

44

ASSESSMENT: Calcaneal varus may be difficult to observe in a standing (weight-bearing) position. Often the weight of the body is enough to cause the calcaneus to appear straight. When weight is removed the varus angulation becomes more prominent. A small degree of varus angulation is normal with the foot in a non-weight-bearing position. Calcaneal varus may also become apparent by looking at the Achilles tendon in relation to a vertical line. If the distal portion of the tendon appears to be curving medially, it may be an indicator of calcaneal varus. A person with calcaneal varus is likely to oversupinate, causing an increasing wear pattern on the outside lateral edge of the shoe. Investigating this shoe wear pattern will often help determine if structural problems exist during normal locomotion.

SUGGESTIONS FOR TREATMENT: This structural problem will often have other components that involve the tibia, knee, femur, or hip joints. It may be difficult address it without addressing more of the comprehensive whole. Massage techniques aimed at reducing the tightness in the inverter muscle group may be helpful. Also, muscular balance between the opposing muscles of the leg that are acting on the foot is likely to contribute. In many instances the best results for changing the nature of this type of structural condition is through some form of movement reeducation. The muscles and other soft-tissues must be taught to move with different patterns of coordination. Orthotics may be used to help encourage the proper alignment of the foot.

(2) CONDITION: CALCANEAL VALGUS

CHARACTERISTICS: This condition is the opposite of calcaneal varus. In this structural problem, the distal portion of the calcaneus is deviating in a lateral direction. Calcaneal valgus will often be present in conjunction with "knock knees" (see condition # 26). It is likely to be present in an individual who overpronates. Tight everter muscles may be present with calcaneal valgus as well. Because of the limitations posed on eversion by the lateral malleolus of the fibula, this condition will usually not be as severe as calcaneal varus.

Figure 4-6
This is a posterior view of the left foot showing calcaneal valgus. The distal portion of the calcaneus is deviating in a lateral direction.

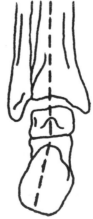

ASSESSMENT: As with calcaneal varus, this condition may be best viewed in a non-weight-bearing position. In this position, the distal portion of the calcaneus (the very base of the heel) will be deviating laterally. The everter muscles of the foot may be tight as well. Since overpronation is a common characteristic with calcaneal valgus a wear pattern will usually be evident on the medial side of the shoe.

SUGGESTIONS FOR TREATMENT: As with calcaneal varus, the whole chain of the lower extremity should be appropriately assessed for involvement in this condition. Massage applications to the everter muscle group may be helpful. Orthotics may also help.

---

(3) CONDITION: SPLAYED FOOT (FALLEN METATARSAL ARCH)

Figure 4-7
Splayed foot.
The metatarsal (transverse) arch has fallen
causing the forefoot and the toes to spread.

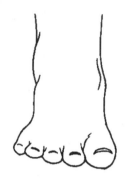

CHARACTERISTICS: The structural support of the foot and its ability to absorb force from weight-bearing is maintained primarily by the crossing arch structures known as the medial and longitudinal arches. When the medial arch is not high enough, the pressure on the forefoot from the weight of the body will cause a fanlike spreading of the metatarsals and phalanges. As the metatarsals and phalanges spread, the foot becomes much less efficient as a shock absorber. This increased amount of shock that is transmitted through the body may eventually show up in other regions such as stress fractures in the tibia.

ASSESSMENT: Assessment of this condition rests primarily on visual inspection. The forefoot will appear wider than normal and the top side of the foot will seem flatter. A proper metatarsal arch will have the top side of the foot appear somewhat rounded from medial to lateral.

SUGGESTIONS FOR TREATMENT: Orthotics will often be recommended to compensate for a fallen metatarsal arch. However, something needs to help the bones of the foot regain the proper arch if at all possible. Certain strengthening exercises, such as towel pulling, may be utilized in order to help strengthen the flexor muscles of the foot. The idea behind this is that it helps create a greater amount of tone in the muscle and develops stamina strength to withstand the long hours of intense loading (body weight) placed on the feet.

---

(4) CONDITION: PES PLANUS (FALLEN LONGITUDINAL ARCH)

CHARACTERISTICS: This is the condition that is commonly referred to as flat feet. The condition of splayed foot above describes a collapse of the metatarsal arch. With splayed foot the forefoot is what is most affected. In pes planus it is the middle section of the longitudinal arch which has fallen. The longitudinal arch is important in withstanding the stress of the body's weight. If the longitudinal arch has collapsed it is likely that other problems affecting the soft-tissues may result. The lack of a sufficient arch often leads to over pronation and medial tibial stress syndrome. Stress fractures are another possible complication caused by the imbalance of stress loading on the foot.

Figure 4-8
Pes planus (fallen longitudinal arch)
The condition commonly known as
"flat feet".

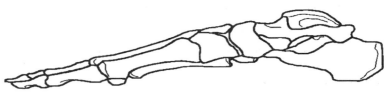

ASSESSMENT: A fallen longitudinal arch is usually visible in a weight-bearing or non-weight-bearing position. In a weight bearing position, the practitioner will notice that it may be difficult to get a finger underneath the most prominent portion of the arch when the person is standing. The bottom surface of the foot will also look relatively "flat". Shoe wear patterns may indicate excessive wear on the medial side as the person is likely to be overpronating as well.

SUGGESTIONS FOR TREATMENT: Orthotics or arch supports of some kind are often used to help compensate for the lack of support from the structure of the foot. There are exercises which are often performed in an effort to strengthen the flexor muscles of the bottom of the foot in order to help maintain the arch. These include trying to pick up objects with the toes or gather up cloth, like a towel, with the toes. Massage applications may be helpful in normalizing muscular balance for the muscles that act on the foot and ankle. The primary problem with pes planus is one of muscular and soft-tissue weakness. Therefore, the best benefits are likely to come from some method of treatment that will strengthen those tissues.

(5) CONDITION: PES CAVUS

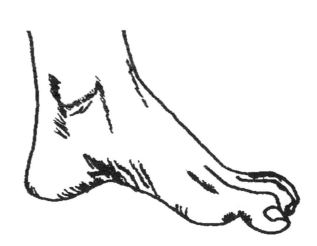

Figure 4-9
Medial view of left foot
showing pes cavus
(high arch)

CHARACTERISTICS: Pes cavus is the opposite of pes planus. It is the foot condition commonly known as a "high arch". In this condition there is a shortening of the plantar fascia and the soft-tissues on the plantar surface of the foot. This functionally raises the longitudinal arch of the foot. When the arch is raised there is an increasing tensile stress placed on the plantar fascia as it absorbs shock during weight-bearing. This increased tensile stress on the plantar fascia will often lead to plantar fascitis or bone spurs developing on the anterior calcaneus.

ASSESSMENT: This condition is best observed in a non-weight-bearing position. The high arch will be readily visible. In certain situations claw toes may accompany pes cavus. Claw toes are characterized by exaggerated flexion of the phalanges as if they are clawing or gripping the ground. The client's toes may not touch the ground when the foot is gently resting on the ground and there may be a prominence to the heads of the metatarsals on the plantar surface of the foot.

SUGGESTIONS FOR TREATMENT: One of the primary perpetuating factors with pes cavus is tightness in the flexor muscles and soft-tissues on the bottom surface of the foot. These tissues will often respond well to massage treatments aimed at lengthening the tissues such as deep stripping techniques on the plantar surface of the foot. Stretching of the calf muscles and flexors of the foot is also likely to help.

---

(6) CONDITION: MORTON'S FOOT

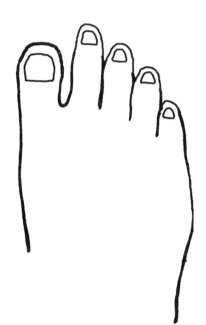

Figure 4-10
Morton's foot
A short hallux in relation to
the second toe

CHARACTERISTICS: Morton's foot is characterized by a short hallux (great toe) in relation to the second toe. This condition is said to be naturally occurring in about 20% of the population. In many individuals it will be totally non-symptomatic and not cause any problems. However, in some people, it may contribute significantly to problems that are experienced in the lower extremity. The shortness of the great toe has a detrimental effect on foot mechanics. The hallux is of prime importance during the push-off phase of the normal gait. If the hallux is shorter, it may not have the length necessary to keep the foot from pronating too far before the push-off. This may be a contributing factor to a number of problems such as plantar fasciitis, or medial tibial stress syndrome.

ASSESSMENT: Morton's foot is easy to detect. Look at the client's feet and see if the second toe is longer than the great toe.

SUGGESTIONS FOR TREATMENT: Morton's foot, because it involves shortness of a bone, will not be corrected by any type of manual therapy. However, some of the soft-tissue stresses that are created by this condition may be addressed through the use of massage, orthotics, or certain stretching, or strength training methods.

(7) CONDITION: HALLUX VALGUS

CHARACTERISTICS: Hallux valgus is a lateral deviation of the distal end of the hallux (great toe). This is usually caused over an extended period of time by wearing shoes with a narrow toe box, such as pointed toe high heels or cowboy boots. As the distal portion of the hallux is driven in a lateral direction, the distal end of the first metatarsal is driven in a medial direction. As the distal head of the first metatarsal moves in a medial direction, a bunion may develop. Bunions will be covered below in condition #8.

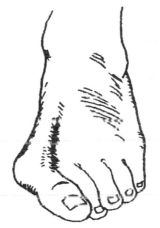

Figure 4-11
Hallux valgus deformity
The distal portion of the hallux is
deviating in a lateral direction

ASSESSMENT: This condition is another one that is clearly visible. Instead of being straight, the distal portion of the hallux will be deviating in a lateral direction just as is illustrated in Figure 4-11. In severe cases, the hallux will not only deviate laterally but it may "ride up" over the second metatarsal.

SUGGESTIONS FOR TREATMENT: This condition has gradually developed by a constant pressure on the hallux over time. It is very difficult to reverse that process because the hallux needs to be pulled in the opposite direction. Some massage techniques may be helpful to loosen up tissues which have become shortened as a result of the hallux position. However, a major realignment of the hallux will need a constant mechanical intervention of some kind.

Common Injury Conditions

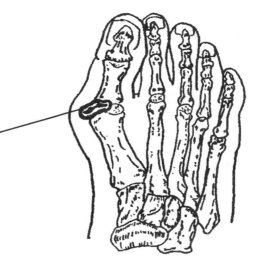

(8) CONDITION: BUNION

Figure 4-12
Bunion on the medial side of the
foot. The bunion is located at the
head of the first metatarsal

CHARACTERISTICS: Bunions develop as a result of hallux valgus deformities. In a hallux valgus deformity the head of the first metatarsal deviates medially as the distal hallux deviates laterally. A callus will form over the protruding head of the first metatarsal. Eventually the bursa over the head of the first metatarsal may become thickened and inflamed. In severe cases this process will culminate in the development of an exostosis or bone spur over the head of the first metatarsal.

ASSESSMENT: Presence of a bunion is determined by visual inspection and palpation. If the client has a hallux valgus deformity, you may automatically suspect that bunions may be present. If there is a thickening of the tissue over the head of the first metatarsal, then callus formation is likely to have begun. If the area is point tender, there may be inflammation of the bursa or a bone spur present.

SUGGESTIONS FOR TREATMENT: Treatment for bunions is virtually identical for that of hallux valgus conditions. Changing the footwear appears to be the most successful treatment.

---

(9) CONDITION: BUNIONETTE (TAILOR'S BUNION)

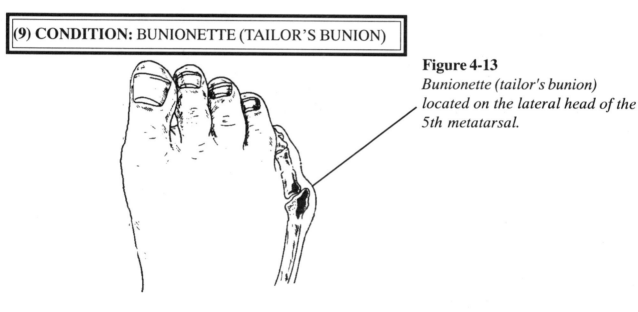

Figure 4-13
Bunionette (tailor's bunion) located on the lateral head of the 5th metatarsal.

CHARACTERISTICS: The bunionette or tailor's bunion has a similar method of development to the bunions caused by hallux valgus deformities. However this bunion develops on the opposite side of the foot at the head of the fifth metatarsal. It is often the result of a splaying or spreading of the metatarsals which will then push the head of the fifth metatarsal against the lateral side of the shoe. It has the same type of callus formation as bunions on the medial side of the foot.

ASSESSMENT: Presence of the bunionette is determined by visual inspection and possible tenderness to palpation. A spreading of the metatarsals along with a history of wearing shoes with a narrow toe box would be contributing factors. Pain may be felt over the head of the fifth metatarsal and it may be protruding slightly.

SUGGESTIONS FOR TREATMENT: Like other bunions, this condition is best managed by a change in footwear.

(10) CONDITION: EXOSTOSIS (BONE SPUR)

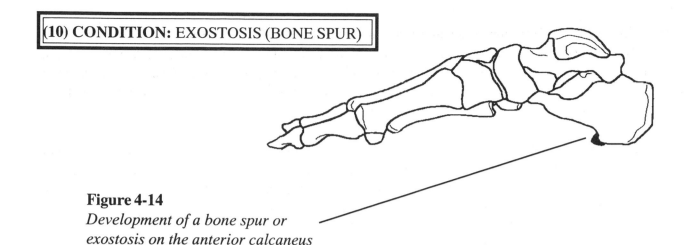

Figure 4-14
*Development of a bone spur or
exostosis on the anterior calcaneus*

CHARACTERISTICS: Bone spurs may develop in many different places in the body. However, the foot is a common location for development of the bone spur. An exostosis often occurs in areas where there is soft-tissue stress on the periosteum of the bone such as at attachment sites of soft-tissue structures. A common site for occurrence of a bone spur is on the anterior portion of the calcaneus at the attachment of the plantar fascia. This is illustrated in Figure 4-14. Bone spurs will develop here because of the added tensile stress on the attachment site. The spur is likely to be tender to the touch and the client will often report pain with activity, especially after having rested for long periods, such as when first arising and walking in the morning.

ASSESSMENT: Certain factors in the history such as overuse of structures that attach in the region of the spur will be common indicators. Tenderness to palpation is also an indicator. In order to confirm the presence of a bone spur, a diagnostic test of bone formation such as an X-Ray or bone scan would be indicated.

SUGGESTIONS FOR TREATMENT: Bone spurs will not be treated directly by massage. Directly applying massage to bone spurs will be counter productive because it is more likely to irritate the tissues further. However, massage can be effectively used to decrease tension on the soft-tissue structures which attach in the region thereby decreasing the amount of irritation from excessive tensile stress.

(11) CONDITION: PLANTAR FASCIITIS

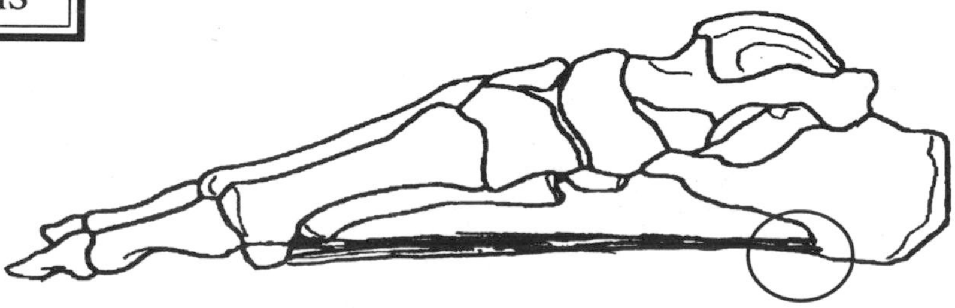

Figure 4-15
*Plantar fasciitis.
The primary region of
pain is circled in the
illustration.*

CHARACTERISTICS: Plantar fasciitis is an overuse condition that arises from irritation and inflammation of the plantar fascia. The plantar fascia has a primary role in maintaining the longitudinal arch of the foot. In a pes cavus (high arch) foot condition, the plantar fascia is shortened and will often cause greater tensile stress on its attachment points as it attempts to absorb shock from the weight of the body. Pain is most often felt at the calcaneal attachment point of the plantar fascia. If this condition is severe, it is likely to involve ossification and development of bone spurs at the attachment site.

ASSESSMENT: Presence of plantar fasciitis is frequently indicated by factors of lower extremity overuse which become evident in the history. People who are actively involved in recreational activities such as running or playing tennis will be likely candidates for this condition. They will usually experience pain along the bottom surface of the foot, especially associated with activity. The pain may be exaggerated when suddenly bearing weight on the foot after a period of prolonged rest, such as when first arising in the morning. There is likely to be point tenderness at the plantar fascia attachment on the anterior calcaneus. There may also be tenderness in the region of the metatarsal heads at the distal plantar fascia attachment sites.

SUGGESTIONS FOR TREATMENT: Plantar fasciitis is most often treated with various conservative measures such as rest, modification of aggravating activities, stretching for the Achilles tendon and flexor muscles of the foot, and cryotherapy or contrast treatments. Massage can be very effective in the management of this condition. Deep transverse friction applied to the plantar fascia will help mobilize this tissue and break fibrous adhesions that are a result of the inflammatory process. Deep longitudinal stripping techniques will also help improve the elongation potential of the fibers. Deep stripping techniques to the tibialis posterior, gastrocnemius, soleus, and other foot and toe flexor muscles will also be helpful. The massage applications are managing the primary complaint and the secondary tissue involvement as well.

---

(12) CONDITION: MORTON'S NEUROMA

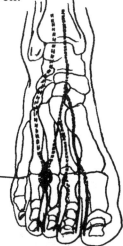

Figure 4-16
Morton's neuroma.
The nerve is pinched
between the heads of
the 3rd and 4th meta-
tarsals.

CHARACTERISTICS: Morton's neuroma is a special type of neuritis. Neuritis is an inflammation or irritation of a nerve. Pain arises in this condition by compression of the junction between the medial and lateral plantar nerves. The junction of these two nerves creates a slightly larger nerve structure between the metatarsal heads . Tight footwear or narrow toe box shoes may cause excessive compression of the nerve junction. Pain and irritation of the nerve result. The pain may be felt in the region of the 3rd and 4th metatarsal heads or it may radiate into the 3rd and 4th toes. The pain is often relieved after removing shoes. Clients may be able to walk pain free barefoot, but then experience discomfort when wearing shoes.

ASSESSMENT: Morton's neuroma is primarily determined by signs and symptoms elicited during the medical history. A history of tight footwear with relief of symptoms after taking off the shoes is a good indicator. The nature and location of the pain will also be indicators. The pain is most often felt at the heads of the 3rd and 4th metatarsals and it is usually a sharp, stinging, type of nerve pain. Certain unique bony formations of the foot in each individual may cause nerve impingement at other metatarsal heads as well.

SUGGESTIONS FOR TREATMENT: This condition is most often managed conservatively with changes in footwear. A wider toe box shoe is recommended. In some instances, orthotics may be called for. If the condition is severe, surgical intervention may be necessary. Direct massage applications to the area are not recommended as a treatment. Since this condition is a result of a mechanically induced impingement from outside forces, there is not much that massage can do to offset that problem. However, some indirect forefoot and metatarsal spreading techniques may decrease compression on the nerve structures. The best approach appears to be footwear changes.

(13) CONDITION: TARSAL TUNNEL SYNDROME

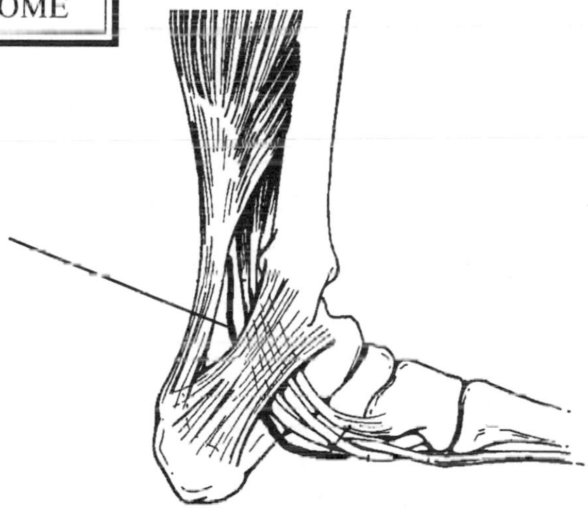

Figure 4-17
Tarsal tunnel syndrome
This is a medial view of the left foot. The posterior tibial nerve is indicated with the line. It travels through the "tunnel" with the adjacent flexor tendons.

CHARACTERISTICS: This is a nerve entrapment condition that happens in the region just posterior and inferior to the medial malleolus of the ankle. It is nowhere near as common as its "cousin" carpal tunnel syndrome in the wrist, but the mechanism of injury is quite similar. The tibial nerve travels posterior and inferior to the medial malleolus as it goes from the ankle down into the foot. As it passes behind the medial malleolus it is in a "tunnel" created by the flexor retinaculum (the "roof"), and the calcaneus and talus (the "floor). In this tunnel it sits between the tendons of the flexor hallucis longus and the flexor digitorum longus muscles. If it is irritated by these structures from overuse or overpronation it will be painful. The client may feel pain in that area or in the area on the bottom surface of the foot supplied by the tibial nerve.

ASSESSMENT: Tarsal tunnel syndrome will become evident mostly through clinical signs and symptoms. The client may report a sharp, shooting pain on the medial side of the ankle while walking. This pain may radiate onto the plantar surface of the foot. Overpronation is another factor which may indicate the possibility of trouble with structures in the tarsal tunnel. Because the sheathed tendons of the tibialis posterior, flexor digitorum longus, and flexor hallucis longus are also in this area, one should be aware that tenosynovitis or tendinitis of these tendons may be the cause for pain in this region. They will also be aggravated by excessive pronation.

SUGGESTIONS FOR TREATMENT: This condition usually involves biomechanical problems of the foot and ankle complex. Reeducation of the gait pattern may be helpful, especially if overpronation is a contributing factor. Irritation of the posterior tibial nerve may be exaggerated by tightness in the flexor muscles that share the tunnel. Longitudinal stripping techniques while actively engaging the tibialis posterior and flexor muscles may enhance fiber elongation and decrease accumulated tension in them. Deep transverse friction applications to the tendons may be called for if tendinitis or tenosynovitis are present. Deep transverse friction should not be performed in the region of the tarsal tunnel if the client feels a sharp shooting pain sensation with the massage application. This indicates that the nerve is being compressed with the friction strokes.

---

(14) CONDITION: RETROCALCANEAL BURSITIS

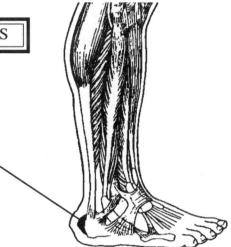

Figure 4-18
Retrocalcaneal bursitis
The line points to the region of
pain and inflammation that
will be present with inflamma-
tion of the bursa.

CHARACTERISTICS: Clients with this condition will present with pain on the back side of the heel. This pain is usually associated with activity and especially with the push-off phase of a walking or running gait. This movement uses the gastrocnemius and soleus muscles. There are actually two bursae behind the calcaneus which may be involved. One is between the Achilles tendon and the calcaneus and the other is between the Achilles tendon and the overlying skin.

ASSESSMENT: The client will often report pain during vigorous activity, especially if it involves running or jumping. There will frequently be pain just anterior to the distal portion of the Achilles tendon, near the insertion point of the Achilles tendon on the calcaneus. This condition can often be differentiated from Achilles tendinitis by squeezing the distal portion of the Achilles tendon above the region of the retrocalcaneal bursa (see the Achilles tendon pinch test in condition # 15). If pain is still felt, one may suspect Achilles tendinitis more than retrocalcaneal bursitis.

SUGGESTIONS FOR TREATMENT: Retrocalcaneal bursitis, like most other bursitis conditions, is best treated with rest and modification of activity. Anti-inflammatory medication or cold applications are also sometimes used. Stretching exercises for the gastrocnemius and soleus are recommended. A heel-lift in the shoe may be used in order to shorten the gastrocnemius and soleus and therefore take tension off the bursa. However, the biomechanical ramifications of lifting one heel may cause muscular imbalance in other areas of the body which could in some cases become a worse secondary problem. Massage applications to the posterior calf muscles are likely to be helpful in reducing the overall tension of these muscles, thereby decreasing the amount of irritation on the bursa.

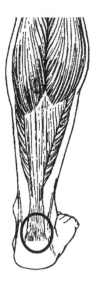

(15) CONDITION: ACHILLES TENDINITIS

Figure 4-19a
Achilles tendinitis
The area circled indicates the
most common site for pain. There
is also likely to be a thickening of
the tendon here.

CHARACTERISTICS: The gastrocnemius and soleus muscles which attach to the calcaneus by way of the Achilles tendon are capable of generating large amounts of force. These muscles are under high demand, especially in various sporting activities which require frequent running or jumping. The distal portion of the Achilles tendon has a very poor blood supply and that is one reason given for the frequent occurrence of tendinitis here. The pain associated with Achilles tendinitis usually occurs in the most distal portion of the tendon.

ASSESSMENT: The client will usually feel pain with activity which subsides with rest. If it is advanced, they may also feel pain with resisted plantar flexion and with passive dorsiflexion which stretches the tendon. Crepitation may be present during active or passive motion. A decreased level of flexibility of the gastrocnemius and soleus are common with this condition. The area of the distal Achilles tendon will likely be tender to palpation. Performing the Achilles tendon pinch test may help determine if it is present.

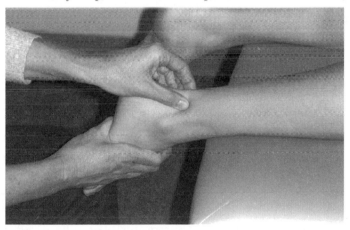

Figure 4-19b
The Achilles tendon
pinch test examining
for Achilles tendinitis.

ACHILLES TENDON PINCH TEST- The therapist will squeeze the sides of the tendon to determine if there is tenderness present. Be careful that the pressure is placed on the sides of the Achilles tendon and not straight down on top of it. If pressure is placed straight down on top of the tendon, pain could be confused with that arising from a retrocalcaneal bursa.

SUGGESTIONS FOR TREATMENT: Like many other tendinitis complaints, this condition is best controlled through rest and modification of activity. However, it is important not to confuse rest with immobilization. Immobilization will often lead to the development of fibrous adhesions. Cold applications and anti-inflammatory medication are often used. As soon as it is tolerable, stretching exercises are helpful. It will be best to perform stretching for the Achilles tendon several times per day. Massage applications to the posterior calf muscles which will reduce the amount of tension in these muscles are indicated. Deep transverse friction as tolerated to the problem area will often help break up fibrous adhesions in the tendon fibers. Cold applications prior to the deep friction will reduce the intensity of the discomfort and reapplying the cold after the treatment will reduce the accelerated metabolic response to the friction.

(16) CONDITION: ACHILLES TENDON RUPTURE

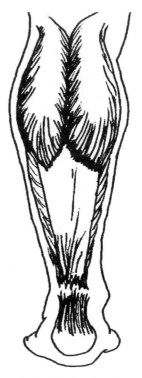

Figure 4-20a
Achilles tendon rupture
This picture illustrates a
complete rupture.

CHARACTERISTICS: There are not many not many muscle/tendon units in the body where you will see a complete rupture. This is a severe injury and the massage therapist will rarely be in a position to see this injury in the acute phase. However, as more massage therapists are becoming involved with athletic events, the chances of them encountering this injury in an acute phase are increased. Complete rupture tends to occur more often in individuals who are not conditioned to high levels of activity, like the "weekend warriors". This condition will frequently occur during athletics when the gastrocnemius and soleus muscles have very high demands put on them.

High levels of repetitive stress loading will frequently weaken the fibrous structures of the Achilles tendon. A sudden overwhelming force may then cause the entire tendon to tear. The rupture will most often happen with either a sudden powerful dorsiflexion of the foot or with a direct blow to the calf muscles while they are contracted. The client will frequently report hearing a loud "popping" sound and have sudden pain which may be accompanied by a severe limitation of plantar flexion.

ASSESSMENT: Since this is an acute injury, getting the client to describe the mechanism of injury as clearly as possible will help the therapist determine the true nature of the problem. A sudden violent dorsiflexion of the foot or blow to the posterior calf is often a causative factor. There will usually be a palpable disruption to the Achilles tendon and the rupture may cause the gastrocnemius and soleus muscles to "bunch up" in the upper (proximal) portion of the leg. The therapist can confirm the presence of an Achilles tendon rupture by performance of the Thompson test.

Figure 4-20b
*The Thompson test
Examining for rupture of
the Achilles tendon.*

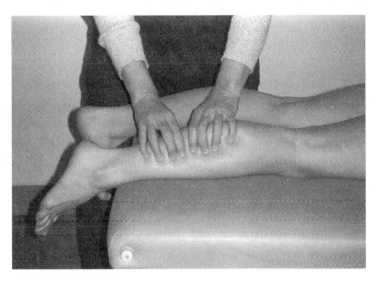

THOMPSON TEST- The client is in a prone position with the knee extended and the foot off the edge of the treatment table. The therapist will squeeze the posterior calf muscles. If no plantar flexion is visible, this is a positive test for an Achilles tendon rupture. If plantar flexion occurs, the test is negative for Achilles tendon rupture.

SUGGESTIONS FOR TREATMENT: If an Achilles tendon rupture is present the client should be immediately referred to a physician for evaluation. Both surgical and nonsurgical approaches are used to treat this condition. The physician will determine which method(s) are appropriate for each circumstance. Nonsurgical approaches involve a prolonged period of immobilization, heel lifts and then a gradual stretching and restrengthening program. Surgical procedures will reattach the torn area and use an appropriate rehabilitation protocol. If a massage therapist is seeing a client who has had a recent Achilles tendon rupture, general massage techniques to the gastrocnemius and soleus may be beneficial in decreasing overall tensile stress on those structures. Any deep friction massage approaches especially at the site of the rupture are not indicated until the rehabilitation has progressed significantly.

(17) CONDITION: LATERAL (INVERSION) ANKLE SPRAINS

Figure 4-21a
*This is a lateral view of the
left foot showing a partially
torn anterior talofibular
ligament from an inversion
ankle sprain. The
calcaneofibular ligament
which is often injured in an
inversion ankle sprain is
also indicated.*

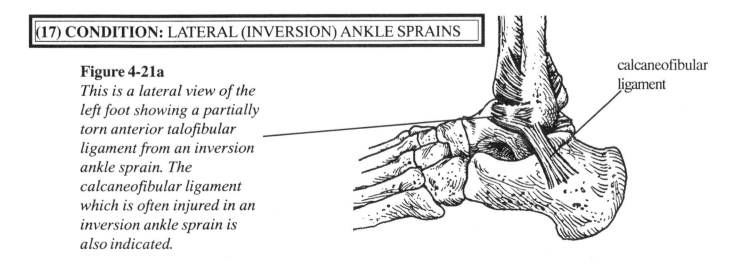

calcaneofibular
ligament

CHARACTERISTICS: In Figure 4-21a you will see a picture of a lateral (inversion) ankle sprain. There are two different types of ankle sprains, lateral (inversion) and medial (eversion). Lateral ankle sprains are far more common. In fact, lateral ankle sprains are one of the most common musculoskeletal injuries. The fibula extends farther distally than the tibia does. This makes the lateral malleolus of the fibula prevent excessive eversion. Because the medial malleolus of the tibia does not extend as far, there is a greater range of motion, and subsequent instability, in inversion. It is the motion of inversion combined with plantar flexion that creates the most frequent lateral ankle sprains. The primary ligament injured in an inversion ankle sprain is the anterior talofibular ligament. Its role is to prevent anterior movement of the talus. More severe inversion sprains will also injure the calcaneofibular ligament.

ASSESSMENT: Lateral ankle sprains occur from an acute injury. The mechanism of injury which the client reports will be an important indicator of which ligaments have been injured. In a lateral ankle sprain the client will usually report twisting the ankle into inversion and then feeling a sudden pain in the region of the lateral ankle. If the motion of plantar flexion was also involved, the likelihood of inversion ankle sprain injury is greater. This injury frequently occurs, for example when someone steps down in a hole. There will be pain and swelling in the region of the lateral malleolus. The injury site will be tender to palpation. Familiarity with the anatomy of the ankle ligament structures will greatly help the practitioner in identifying which structures have been injured. Disruption of the anterior talofibular ligament can also be determined by use of the ankle drawer sign.

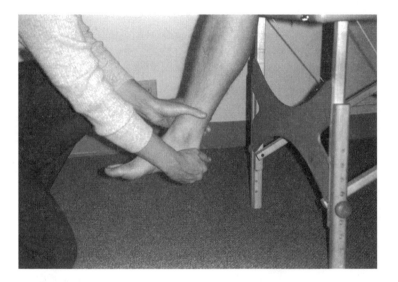

Figure 4-21b
The Ankle drawer sign examining for instability from a lateral/inversion ankle sprain.

ANKLE DRAWER SIGN- This test is designed to determine the integrity of the anterior talofibular ligament. The client's leg is suspended off the end of the treatment table. The practitioner will stabilize the foot with one hand while pushing in a posterior direction on the distal tibia with the other hand. If movement occurs, this indicates an instability of the anterior talofibular ligament (an anterior movement of the talus in relation to the fibula).

SUGGESTIONS FOR TREATMENT: Ankle sprains are best treated in the initial stage with the RICE acronym (Rest, Ice, Compression, and Elevation). Once the severity of the ligament sprain has been determined, the course of treatment can be further defined. A severe ligament sprain may warrant surgical intervention. However, most ligament sprains can be managed by conservative means.

Swelling will usually be present in the area for quite a while after the acute phase of the injury has subsided. ROM exercises, stretching of the muscles around the ankle joint, and proprioceptive exercises using a wobble (B.A.P.S.) board are recommended as soon as it is tolerable. Drawing letters of the alphabet with the toes in the air with the foot in a non-weight bearing position is often used as an exercise to help return movement in all planes. Any movement exercises should be done within the clients comfort range. Massage applications can be very beneficial for the healing of ankle sprains. General applications to the muscles of the calf will help reduce the continuation of protective spasms which may have begun at the onset of the injury. Special attention to the peroneal muscles of the calf is indicated for lateral ankle sprains. These muscles will help enhance the stability of the ankle to compensate for the injured ligament(s). Once the acute phase of the injury has subsided, deep transverse friction to the injured ligaments combined with ROM will enhance the proper alignment of scar tissue for the most functional repair of the injury site.

(18) CONDITION: MEDIAL (EVERSION) ANKLE SPRAINS

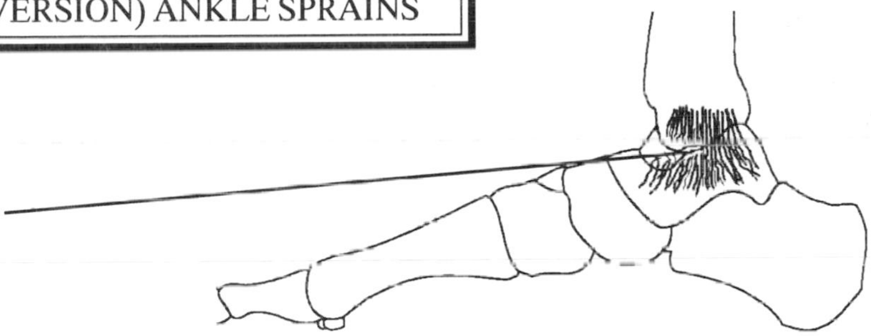

Figure 4-22
Medial view of right foot showing injury to the deltoid ligament from a medial/eversion ankle sprain.

CHARACTERISTICS: Although medial ankle sprains are far less common, when they do occur, the mechanism of injury will often cause them to be quite severe. They sometimes involve avulsion fractures of the distal tibia. Eversion or medial ankle sprains will injure the deltoid ligament which is actually composed of several smaller ligaments. Pain and swelling will be present near the medial malleolus with an eversion sprain.

ASSESSMENT: Medial ankle sprains will have a history of sudden eversion stress to the foot/ankle complex. There will be point tenderness and swelling present around the underside of the medial malleolus. There may also be a sense of instability around the ankle joint. If the deltoid ligament was involved in an avulsion injury the condition is likely to be more painful and more severe.

SUGGESTIONS FOR TREATMENT: See the description listed for inversion ankle sprains. The methods of treatment will be very similar with the major difference only being the site of injury.

(19) CONDITION: SHIN SPLINTS

CHARACTERISTICS: Shin Splints is a catchall term that may refer to a variety of overuse problems affecting the leg. There are two different types of shin splints. Anterior-lateral (AL) shin splints are usually attributed to overuse of the dorsiflexor muscles such as the tibialis anterior, extensor digitorum longus, and extensor hallucis longus. The overuse will frequently happen as a result of excessive eccentric loading on the dorsiflexors. Eccentric loading to the dorsiflexors can happen during running or if, for example, the client has been walking or running downhill for significant distances. What determines a significant distance will depend on what that person's body has been conditioned to.

The second type of shin splints is posterior-medial (PM). This condition is sometimes referred to in the medical literature as medial tibial stress syndrome (MTSS). This is an overuse problem but MTSS is caused by overuse to the muscular structures that resist pronation, primarily tibialis posterior. Flat feet (pes planus), inadequate footwear, overpronation, running on hard surfaces, or improper biomechanical function of the foot or leg may all lead to MTSS. As the tibialis posterior attempts to resist excessive pronation it becomes over stressed leading to inflammation and irritation along its proximal attachment sites on the tibia, fibula, and interosseous membrane.

Figure 4-23a
Anterior view of left leg. Regions of pain with anterior/ lateral shin splints and medial tibial stress syndrome.

region of pain in MTSS

region of pain in anterior/lateral shin splints

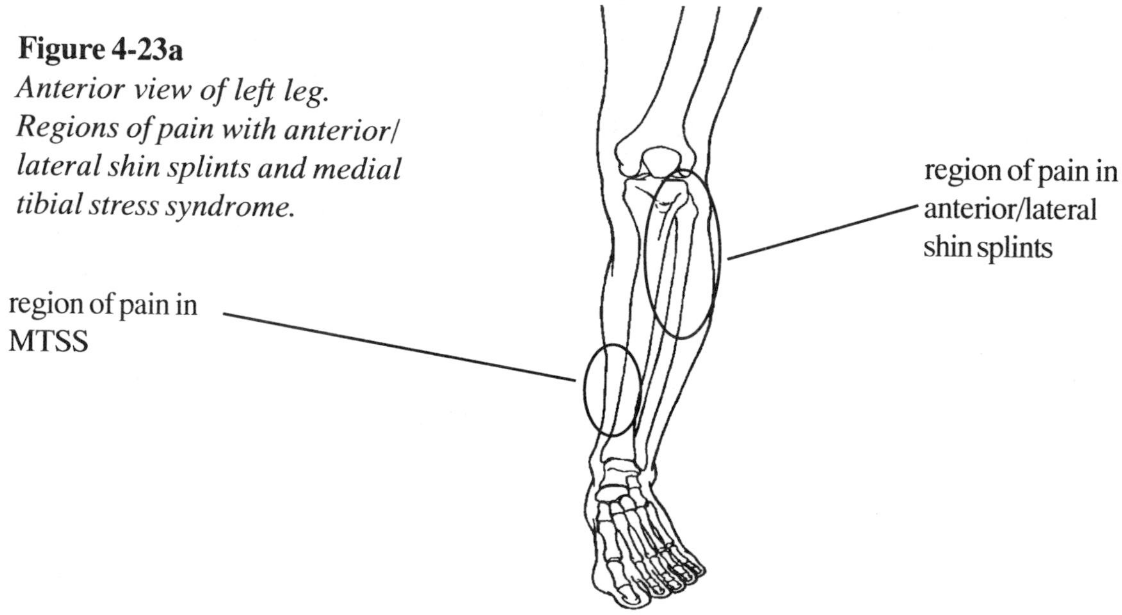

ASSESSMENT: Because shin splints is a poorly defined catchall term, it is hard to say what actually defines them. In an attempt to clarify what might be present, this text will discuss assessment of shin splints as either 1) overuse problem affecting the dorsiflexor muscles (AL shin splints) or 2) overuse problem affecting primarily the tibialis posterior muscle (MTSS). One of the most important factors when assessing the presence or severity of shin splints is to rule out more severe conditions such as compartment syndrome or stress fractures. See the information on these conditions in this section.

AL shin splints can most often be determined by several factors. A history which indicates recent overuse will be important. The client with AL shin splints may report pain all along the lateral border of the tibia. This whole region may be sore because the muscle attachment along the periosteum is quite broad. The periosteum is the most pain sensitive tissue in the body, so overuse and tensile stress is frequently painful. The client may have pain on resisted dorsiflexion. If the client maintains a position of dorsiflexion of the foot and the therapist presses on the tibialis anterior while the client maintains this contraction, pain may be produced if AL shin splints are present.

MTSS, like the AL shin splints, will often be determined by a history of recent overuse. These factors along with flat feet, overpronation, or recent changes in activity may indicate MTSS. With MTSS, pain will be felt on the distal, medial portion of the tibia, usually in the most distal 1/3 of thetibia. The distal portion of the tibia, and often the whole attachment region of the tibialis posterior, will be tender to palpation. Pressing along the medial border of the tibia may cause pain if MTSS is present. Pain is usually diffuse

60

and spread over a wider area with MTSS than with a stress fracture. That is one way to distinguish the possibility of MTSS versus a stress fracture.

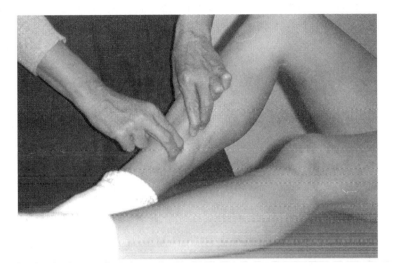

Figure 4-23b
Pressing the medial border of the tibia to examine for MTSS

SUGGESTIONS FOR TREATMENT: Both forms of shin splints (AL and MTSS) are most often treated with conservative measures. Modification of activities and rest will usually allow this condition to subside without other intervention. However, the day to day activities of walking and movement may cause the condition to persist. Also, the client may be involved with some type of activity (dance, running, etc.) that they do not want to quit. In addition to modifying activities, massage applications can get very good results with both these types of conditions. Friction applications, although not comfortable, will often help reduce fibrous adhesions that may have developed along the tendinous fibers. Massage applications that are performed in conjunction with active and passive movements are also likely to benefit.

There have been discussions in the massage community about not working away from the tibia on shin splints because it "pulls the muscle away from the bone". Although many people subscribe to this theory, sound evidence for it does not exist. It is likely that this concept has developed more out of imagery than actual occurrences. Tendons are incredibly resistant to tensile stress. Although irritated in these conditions, and during massage strokes, they are rarely subjected to the amount of force that would cause tendon avulsions. The tensile stress on the tendon fibers of the muscles during normal walking are much greater than that applied with the fingers during massage. Therefore it seems highly unlikely that a manual treatment would cause a tendon avulsion.

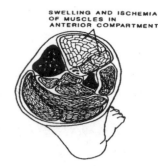

SWELLING AND ISCHEMIA
OF MUSCLES IN
ANTERIOR COMPARTMENT

ANTERIOR COMPARTMENT SYNDROME

Figure 4-24
*Cross section of the leg
just below the knee joint.
Notice the swelling in the
anterior compartment.
(Illustration courtesy of
Educational Graphics)*

CHARACTERISTICS: Illustrated in Figure 4-24 are different muscular compartments of the lower leg. There are fascial planes or walls that separate each of these different muscular compartments. A traumatic blow or chronic overuse may cause swelling in the compartments. This will happen most often in the anterior compartment. The anterior compartment contains the tibialis anterior muscle, the extensor hallucis longus, and extensor digitorum longus muscles, as well as the deep peroneal nerve and the anterior tibial artery and veins. When swelling happens within the compartment as a result of a traumatic blow or chronic overuse, it may impede the flow of blood in the artery or veins, or it may impinge the deep peroneal nerve. This may cause pain and discomfort that is associated with activity and which decreases with rest. Impingement of the deep peroneal nerve may also lead to diminished function of the dorsiflexor muscles (tibialis anterior, extensor digitorum longus, and extensor hallucis longus). This diminished function may show up as the neurological deficit called "drop foot". Drop foot is characterized by a lack of dorsiflexion in the normal gait pattern so that when the foot is picked up off the ground it may drag and contact the ground in a more plantar flexed position than its normal dorsiflexed position.

ASSESSMENT: Anterior compartment syndrome is characterized by a history of a traumatic blow to the anterior shin or by chronic overuse. If the condition is of a chronic nature, pain will be most associated with activity and will diminish with rest. The client may also complain of the foot or toes being cold or feeling that they do not have good control of their foot. Pain, dysfunction, or paresthesia of the dorsiflexor muscles will be an indicator of neurological impingement. It is important to remember that you may see neurological or vascular signs or both. If the condition is not severe, you might not see either readily. In this instance it is easy to confuse compartment syndrome with shin splints. The client with compartment syndrome will report that the pain is a deep and cramping type of pain. Muscle weakness may also be present. Presence of compartment syndrome is best confirmed by taking an intracompartmental pressure reading and comparing that with the unaffected side or with changes that occur as a result of activity. However, this requires specialized equipment.

SUGGESTIONS FOR TREATMENT: Conservative forms of treatment such as ice, rest, modification of activity, and stretching are often employed in an effort to treat compartment syndrome. However, if this condition is severe, it is frequently treated with a surgical procedure called a fasciotomy where an incision is made in the fascial compartmental wall in order to relieve the excess pressure. Massage applications may be helpful in reducing compartmental pressures by assisting in the movement of local tissue fluids. However, massage should not be performed when the compartment is in an inflamed condition.

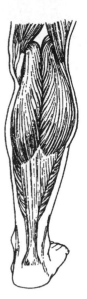

(21) CONDITION: MUSCLE CRAMPING (CALF)

Figure 4-25
The triceps surae muscle group composed of the gastrocnemius and soleus. This muscle group is the most common site for muscle cramping.

CHARACTERISTICS: The calf is the region most frequently affected with muscle cramps. A muscle cramp is a sustained involuntary muscular spasm. There are several different theories about what causes muscle cramping. It has been attributed to factors such as salt deprivation, potassium imbalance, and local tissue dehydration. It will commonly occur in athletic activity following particularly strenuous bouts of exercise. It may also occur if a muscle is immobilized in a shortened position immediately following chronic exertion.

ASSESSMENT: It is difficult to miss a muscle cramp. Although they will usually be associated with recent athletic activity, the massage therapist may have a client suddenly have a calf cramp when on the treatment table. This may happen if the client has been prone for a long period of time with the feet fully plantar flexed (this happens in a prone position without a bolster, pillow, or support under the ankles. The client will report severe pain or discomfort (usually in the calf or flexor muscles of the foot or toes). Pain will be increased with pressure on the muscles and passive stretching will also cause an increase in pain.

SUGGESTIONS FOR TREATMENT: Although massage is often recommended for a cramp, it does not appear as effective as some methods of stretching. Stretching methods such as PNF which incorporate reciprocal inhibition or contraction of an antagonist muscle will often interrupt the neurological cycle which is perpetuating the spasm.

(22) CONDITION: STRESS FRACTURE

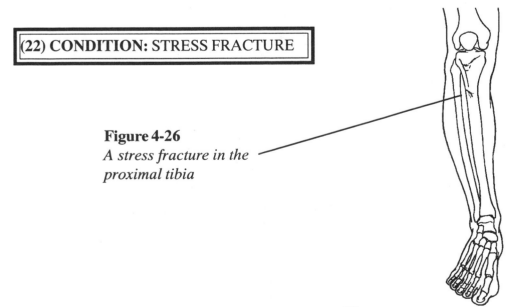

Figure 4-26
A stress fracture in the proximal tibia

63

CHARACTERISTICS: A stress fracture is an overuse condition that develops as a result of repetitive stress loading on the bone. It occurs most often in the weight bearing bones such as the tibia, but it can also occur in a non-weight bearing bone such as the fibula. A stress fracture may at first be dismissed as being shin splints. However, if left untreated it may become a very problematic chronic injury. The client will usually complain of pain that is associated with the activity which subsides with rest.

ASSESSMENT: Factors in the history which point to chronic overuse or repetitive stress loading on hard surfaces will be indicators of a stress fracture. A stress fracture can often be differentiated from a soft-tissue musculoskeletal condition by the nature and location of the pain. While a musculoskeletal condition often has diffuse pain which may be increased with engagement of the muscle/tendon unit in a manual resistive test, a stress fracture presents with a smaller localized area of pain. Tapping on the bone or placing a vibrating tuning fork on the bone may also produce pain. This would not be likely to cause pain in a musculoskeletal condition. X-rays may be used to determine a stress fracture, but they are often inconclusive. The best method of determining the presence of a stress fracture is with a bone scan. A bone scan will show the region of increased metabolic activity in the bone that is characteristic of a fracture healing site.

SUGGESTIONS FOR TREATMENT: The most effective way of addressing stress fractures is through rest and modification of activity. Because it is a bone fracture, time and reduction of the aggravating forces will be most important. Some modalities, such as electrical stimulation, have been used with some success in speeding the healing of fracture sites. Massage applications may be helpful in normalizing biomechanical stresses in the region of the stress fracture.

---

(23) CONDITION: DORSIFLEXOR TENOSYNOVITIS (LACE BITE)

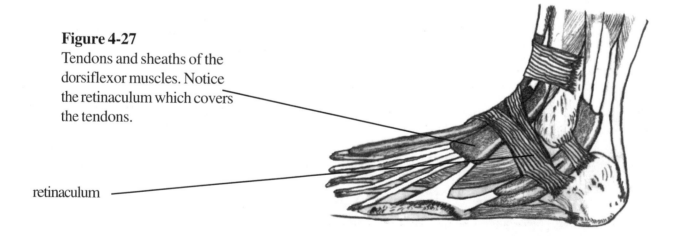

Figure 4-27
Tendons and sheaths of the dorsiflexor muscles. Notice the retinaculum which covers the tendons.

retinaculum

CHARACTERISTICS: The tendons for the dorsiflexor muscles travel under a soft tissue retinaculum at the ankle joint. They must be free to move underneath that retinaculum. If there is constant pressure on the top side of the foot the dorsiflexor tendons will be inhibited in their action. This may cause a roughening or

ASSESSMENT: Lace bite will generally be tender to direct pressure on the tendon sheaths. It is likely that there will be tenderness on the dorsal surface of the foot with resisted dorsiflexion. A history that involves wearing tight shoes or some type of footwear that may "bind" across the top of the foot is a common indicator.

SUGGESTIONS FOR TREATMENT: Lace bite can be treated like other tenosynovitis conditions. Deep transverse friction on the offending tendons is used to break up adhesion between the tendon and its sheath. Massage applications to the dorsiflexor muscles are used to help them reduce tension on the tendons. Changing the footwear, which may be the primary problem, is highly indicated.

(24) CONDITION: MUSCLE STRAINS

CHARACTERISTICS: Acute overloading of musculotendinous structures in the leg, ankle and foot will lead to muscle strains. They may happen in several different locations. Strains to the peroneal muscles, for example, will often happen in conjunction with a lateral ankle sprain as those muscles attempt to resist inversion.

ASSESSMENT: Knowledge of anatomy will be crucial in determining the presence of muscle strains. These conditions may have a number of symptoms depending on their severity. See the section in the beginning of the book on muscle strains for a more complete description of the differences between the various grades of strain. Determination of muscle pain or weakness may be based on the use of various manual resistive tests which isolate that muscle. Manual resistive tests for the four single plane movements of the foot and ankle are included at the beginning of this chapter:

SUGGESTIONS FOR TREATMENT: Any discussion of the treatment of muscle strains must be considered relative to the degree of the strain. For instance, the method of treatment for a grade 1 strain will be different from that of a severe grade 3 strain. In most instances muscle strains will be treated with rest from the offending activity, some type of anti-inflammatory treatment, stretching in the post-acute phase, and gradual strengthening as the injury repair progresses. Massage applications such as deep transverse friction are quite effective in helping to create a functional scar that is strong, yet pliable enough not to impair the proper use of the tissue. Massage is also very helpful during the rehabilitative phase to decrease muscle spasm which may have occurred immediately after the injury and is preventing the proper biomechanical balance from returning.

(25) CONDITION: NEUROMUSCULAR PAIN

CHARACTERISTICS: Any muscle in the body is capable of holding an increased level of neurological activity and maintaining a spasm. The spasm of that muscle will then lead to increased pain and disturbed biomechanical function. Muscle spasm can be perpetuated by various stimuli including chemicals like caffeine, certain medications, myofascial trigger points, or emotional stress. The pain may be relieved by rest, but simple activities of daily living will often cause the pain to resurface. These conditions are some of the most frequent problems encountered by any health care practitioner who works with the musculoskeletal system. They may often be dismissed as irrelevant or inconsequential by some practitioners, but many clinicians are now admitting the importance of these muscular problems has been overlooked in our health care system.

ASSESSMENT: The muscles will frequently be painful in certain areas to palpation, may demonstrate a decreased range of motion, and may be somewhat painful on a resisted isometric contraction or stretch. They may contain painful myofascial trigger points which refer pain or other autonomic phenomena to remote areas. Chronic overuse, postural or biomechanical imbalances which are evident through the history may be indicating factors. See the sections above for references on manual resistive tests and range of motion testing for selected muscles of the leg, ankle, and foot.

SUGGESTIONS FOR TREATMENT: These conditions respond favorably to massage applications. Since muscular spasm is a primary component of these conditions, a technique like massage that is highly effective in addressing muscular spasm is very effective in reducing the complaint. If the condition arises from poor postural or biomechanical function, movement reeducation is very helpful, and in most cases necessary, as an adjunctive treatment.

Quick Reference for Conditions of the Foot, Ankle, & Leg

REGION OF PAIN	ONSET	POSSIBLE CAUSE	REF.
MEDIAL SIDE OF 1ST METATARSAL HEAD	CHRONIC	BUNION	8
LATERAL SIDE OF 5TH METATARSAL HEAD	CHRONIC	BUNIONETTE (TAILOR'S BUNION)	9
VARIOUS LOCATIONS (BASE OF ANTERIOR CALCANEUS)	CHRONIC	BONE SPUR EXOSTOSIS	10
PLANTAR SURFACE OF FOOT BASE OF ANTERIOR CALCANEUS	CHRONIC	PLANTAR FASCITIS	11
BETWEEN 3RD AND 4TH METATARSALS ALSO INTO 3RD OR 4TH TOES	CHRONIC	MORTON'S NEUROMA	12
MEDIAL ANKLE REGION DOWN ALONG MEDIAL SIDE OF FOOT TO PLANTAR SURFACE	CHRONIC	TARSAL TUNNEL SYNDROME	13
POSTERIOR SIDE OF CALCANEUS	CHRONIC	RETROCALCANEAL BURSITIS	14
DISTAL PORTION OF ACHILLES TENDON	CHRONIC	ACHILLES TENDINITIS	15
ACHILLES TENDON FROM MUSCLE-TENDON JUNCTION TO CALCANEUS	ACUTE	ACHILLES TENDON RUPTURE	16
LATERAL SIDE OF ANKLE	ACUTE	LATERAL ANKLE SPRAIN	17
MEDIAL SIDE OF ANKLE	ACUTE	MEDIAL ANKLE SPRAIN	18
ANTERIOR/LATERAL SHIN REGION	CHRONIC	ANTERIOR/LATERAL SHIN SPLINTS	19
MEDIAL SIDE OF DISTAL TIBIA	CHRONIC	MEDIAL TIBIAL STRESS SYNDROME	19
ANTERIOR REGION OF LEG	ACUTE OR CHRONIC	ANTERIOR COMPARTMENT SYNDROME	20
POSTERIOR CALF/PLANTAR SURFACE OF FOOT	ACUTE	MUSCLE CRAMPING	21
VARIOUS LOCATIONS/COMMONLY ON DISTAL PORTION OF TIBIA	CHRONIC	STRESS FRACTURE	22
DORSAL SURFACE OF FOOT	CHRONIC	DORSIFLEXOR TENOSYNOVITIS	23
ANY MUSCLE	ACUTE OR CHRONIC	MUSCLE STRAIN	24
ANY MUSCLE	CHRONIC	NEUROMUSCULAR PAIN	25

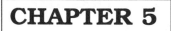

KNEE AND THIGH CONDITIONS

SPECIAL TERMS AND CONCEPTS

1) MOVIE SIGN- is a name given for a symptom of pain in the knees that happens as a result of maintaining the knee in flexion for prolonged periods such as when watching a movie in a theater. A person with a positive movie sign will experience pain on arising (from the prolonged flexion position) that will gradually dissipate after they start moving around.

2) VMO- is an acronym for vastus medialis obliquus. This is the most distal portion of the vastus medialis muscle. The fibers run in an oblique inferior and medial direction. This muscle is chiefly responsible for offsetting the lateral pull on the patella by the vastus lateralis. The lateral pull on the patella can be exaggerated if the Q angle (see the discussion of the Q angle in the structural and postural deviations section) is large because the distal portion of the femur is at a greater medial deviation. This medial deviation of the distal femur causes the patella to track closer to the lateral femoral condyle than straight in the groove between the condyles. If the VMO is not of sufficient strength, it will not be able to offset these structural stresses and various patellar tracking problems may result such as chondromalacia.

OVERVIEW OF COMMON SINGLE PLANE MOVEMENTS OF THE KNEE

Flexion- A movement at the knee which decreases the joint angle so the lower leg and the thigh come closer together. Normal flexion should be approximately 160° or when the muscles of the calf meet and press against the hamstring muscles of the thigh. The primary muscles used in flexion are:
>   **Biceps Femoris**
>   **Semimembranosus**
>   **Semitendinosus**
>   **Gastrocnemius**
>   **Plantaris**
>   **Popliteus**

Extension- The reference position of anatomical position is considered full extension. Extension may also be used to describe the return to the anatomical reference position from any degree of flexion. Normal range of extension is 180°. Some individuals can move the knee slightly past the full extension position while in a standing position. This is often referred to as hyperextension of the knees. Hyperextension in a standing position is also known as genu recurvatum (see the discussion of genu recurvatum in the structural and postural deviations section). The primary muscles used in extension are:

Rectus Femoris
Vastus Medialis
Vastus Lateralis
Vastus Intermedius

Active Range of Motion Tests

Active range of motion tests for the knee will focus on the two single plane movements described above. If specific information is desired about particular muscle action during active range of motion tests, be aware of what muscles are actually being used. A review of the discussion of concentric and eccentric muscle contractions will be helpful. For example, an active range of motion evaluation for the knee can be performed in a standing position where full flexion and extension are both permitted. However, due to the position of the body and the influence of gravity, only the hamstring muscles are engaged - concentrically during the flexion movements and eccentrically during the extension movements.

Passive Range of Motion Tests

The practitioner should pay particular attention to end-feels when performing passive range of motion tests. Also, because of the prevalence of ligament injuries at the knee, it is important to compare findings of active versus passive range of motion tests in order to determine which structures are primarily involved.

The end-feel for knee extension is a short tissue stretch (ligament stretch). It may feel almost like a bone-to-bone end-feel. Note that this assumes that the client's hip is not in a position of flexion. If the client's hip is flexed, the end-feel is likely to be a true tissue stretch as the limitation is produced by the resistance of the hamstring muscle/tendon unit.

The end-feel for knee flexion is that of soft-tissue approximation in a knee that has normal range of motion. If motion in the knee is limited by quadriceps tightness, the end-feel will be that of tissue stretch as the quadriceps muscle/tendon units resist the motion.

Manual Resistive Tests

The next section includes illustrations and descriptions of manual resistive tests for the two single plane movements of the knee. Remember that each of these movements can be performed in either of the two ways described earlier to perform manual resistive tests.

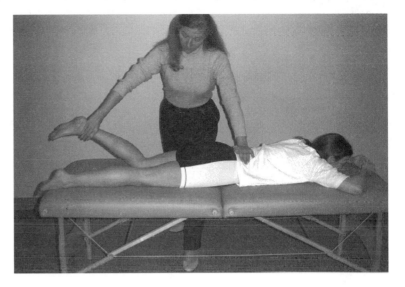

Figure 5-1
Resisted knee flexion

The client is in a prone position on the treatment table with the knee in a position of partial flexion. The therapist places one hand on the lumbar region for stabilization and the other hand on the posterior side of the distal tibia. The client will be instructed to hold the leg in this position as the therapist attempts to move the leg into extension.

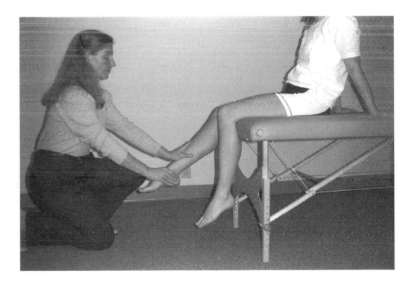

Figure 5-2
Resisted Knee Extension

The client is in a seated position on the edge of the treatment table with the knee in a position of partial extension. The therapist will place both hands on the distal portion of the tibia. The client will be instructed to hold the leg in this position while the therapist attempts to move the leg into flexion.

Structural and Postural Deviations

---
(26) CONDITION: GENU VALGUM

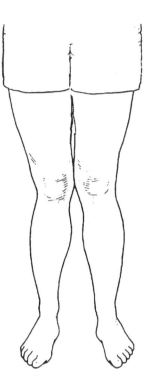

Figure 5-3
Genu valgum.
Lateral deviation of the
distal portion of the tibia.
The condition known as
"knock knees".

CHARACTERISTICS: Genu valgum is a structural condition of the knees that is commonly referred to as "knock-knees". Valgus angulation refers to the lateral deviation of the distal portion of a bony segment. At the knees, the bony segment being referred to is the tibia. In this structural condition, the distal portion of the tibia deviates laterally which makes the proximal portion more medial. This causes the knees to come together. Additional stress will be placed on the soft-tissue structures as they attempt to compensate for the altered mechanical alignment. Genu valgum often occurs in conjunction with a large Q angle (see the discussion of Q angles below).

ASSESSMENT: Genu valgum should be assessed from the front or the rear. If it is present, the thighs will come together and the knees will appear overly close to each other. A line along the tibia will indicate that the distal portion of the tibia is further lateral than the medial portion. In a normal alignment the tibia should be vertical.

SUGGESTIONS FOR TREATMENT: Mechanical and postural reeducation is important for this condition. This alignment of the knees is likely to put additional tensile stress on the adductors and the medial collateral ligament of the knee and additional compressive stress on the lateral meniscus. Massage and stretching can be used to enhance the mechanical balance of all the lower extremity muscles. Because this condition develops over time and will often be an integral part of the entire lower extremity alignment (i.e. it may be caused by calcaneal valgus), the best results will be obtained with an approach which incorporates the entire kinetic chain.

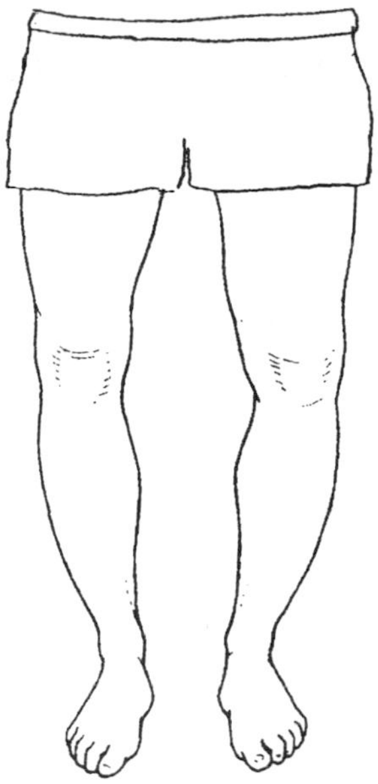

Figure 5-4
Genu varum.
Medial deviation of the
distal portion of the tibia.
The condition known as
"bowlegged".

CHARACTERISTICS: Genu varum is commonly referred to as "bowlegs". It is the opposite of genu valgum. In this condition the distal portion of the tibia will deviate medially. A lateral angulation of the distal femur will cause a lateral angulation of the proximal tibia. The distal tibia will then angle medially. As with genu valgum, stresses will be placed on the soft-tissues as they attempt to compensate for the improper weight-bearing alignment of the bones.

ASSESSMENT: This condition is best assessed from the front or rear. There will be considerable space between the legs and the person will have the characteristic "bowleg" stance. Additional wear is likely to be seen on the outside edge of the shoe.

SUGGESTIONS FOR TREATMENT: This structural alignment will put additional tensile stress on the iliotibial band and the lateral collateral ligament, and additional compressive stress on the medial meniscus of the knee. The additional tensile stress on the iliotibial band may be the cause for ITB friction syndrome (see the description later in this chapter). Massage applications may be beneficial to all the muscles of the lower extremity in order to enhance biomechanical balance. However, just as with genu valgum, a postural reeducation is really necessary in order to make a lasting change.

(28) CONDITION: GENU RECURVATUM

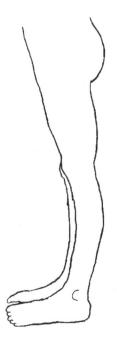

Figure 5-5
Genu recurvatum
The condition commonly
referred to as "locked knees".

CHARACTERISTICS: People often refer to this as the position of "locked" knees. The knee is past full extension and a degree of ligamentous laxity allows the knees to go into hyperextension. In most cases, since this will only be present in a standing position, it is not problematic for knee mechanics. However, if a person is standing for long periods, the genu recurvatum tends to also exaggerate anterior pelvic tilt (see condition # 43) which increases problems in the low back region.

ASSESSMENT: This condition is best assessed from a lateral view. When the knees are in full extension, they should be vertical. If they move past vertical into hyperextension, there will be slight curvature to the whole lower extremity that is concave in an anterior direction.

SUGGESTIONS FOR TREATMENT: Genu recurvatum is usually the result of genetically inherited ligamentous laxity. As mentioned above, it rarely causes problems during active knee movement. However, for long periods of standing it can be a problem causing knee stress or low back problems. The most effective way to alleviate it is through postural awareness and reeducation in the standing position.

(29) CONDITION: EXCESSIVE Q ANGLE

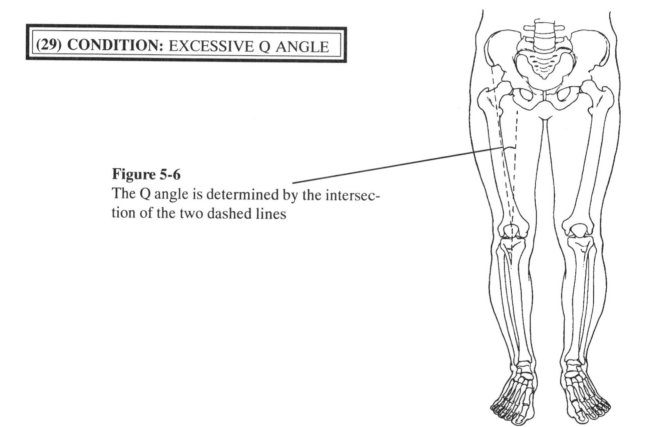

Figure 5-6
The Q angle is determined by the intersection of the two dashed lines

CHARACTERISTICS: The Q angle (quadriceps angle) is a measurement that is used to determine characteristics of alignment that will affect knee mechanics. The angle is based on the approximate direction of pull of the quadriceps muscle group. The Q angle is described by the angle formed between two imaginary lines. The first is created by drawing a line from the tibial tuberosity through the midpoint of the patella. The second is formed by drawing a line from the ASIS through the midpoint of the patella. The angle formed between these two lines is the Q angle. An excessively large Q angle (more than 15^0 in men or 20^0 in women) is often referred to as malicious malalignment syndrome because of the many problems with knee mechanics and patellar tracking that it causes. A large Q angle is often a factor in a number of the conditions that will be discussed in the common injury section such as patello-femoral pain syndrome and chondromalacia.

ASSESSMENT: The Q angle can be measured by using strings between the anatomical landmarks described above. However, it is more often used as a general descriptive term applied to the angulation of the femur without taking exact measurements. Notice that a wider pelvis will make the Q angle larger.

~NO

SUGGESTIONS FOR TREATMENT: The Q angle is a genetically determined aspect of skeletal structure and can not be altered. It is, however, an important characteristic to keep in mind when addressing a variety of knee problems.

Common Injury Conditions

(30) CONDITION: ANTERIOR CRUCIATE LIGAMENT SPRAIN

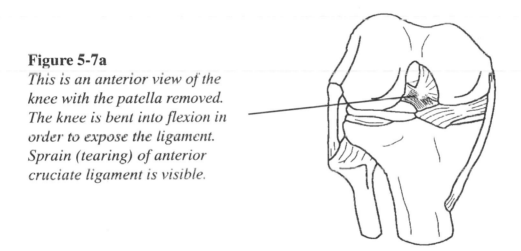

Figure 5-7a
This is an anterior view of the knee with the patella removed. The knee is bent into flexion in order to expose the ligament. Sprain (tearing) of anterior cruciate ligament is visible.

CHARACTERISTICS: The anterior cruciate ligament (ACL) is one of four primary ligaments which stabilize the knee. There are additional accessory ligaments but four are responsible for most of the structural stability in the knee. The ACL prevents anterior movement of the tibia in relation to the femur. It also provides some resistance to medial rotation of the knee joint (actually medial rotation of the tibia). Although the primary role of the ligament is preventing anterior movement of the tibia it is most often injured with rotational stress to the knee. Rotary stress to the knee frequently happens in various activities, especially in athletics. The most common mechanism of rotary stress to the knee is when a person plants a foot and then turns the body.

ASSESSMENT: A client with an injured ACL will usually report a movement such as those described above which led to the injury. He/she may report hearing a loud pop that was immediately followed by serious pain and discomfort. Although the anterior cruciate ligament is deep within the knee, the client may also report pain in the medial joint line region. That is because injuries to the ACL are often associated with injuries to other joint structures. The ACL is part of a group of three tissues commonly injured together known as the "Terrible Triad". They consist of the ACL, the medial collateral ligament (MCL), and medial meniscus. There are several methods used to test integrity of the ACL. One of the most commonly relied upon is the Lachman test.

75

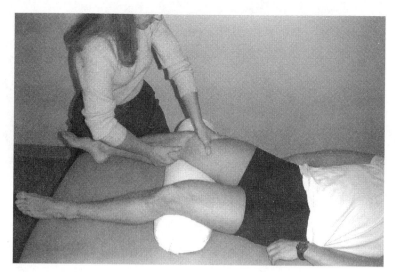

Figure 5-7b
The Lachman test for injury to the anterior cruciate ligament

LACHMAN TEST- The Lachman test is performed with the client in a supine position. The knee is in a position between full extension and 30° of flexion. The practitioner grasps the proximal tibia with the inferior hand and grasps the distal femur with the superior hand. The practitioner will then attempt to pull the proximal tibia forward with the inferior hand while the superior hand stabilizes the femur and feel if there is any movement. A positive sign for ACL disruption is a soft or "mushy" end-feel to the movement. The practitioner may also notice a change in slope to the infrapatellar tendon. The Lachman test is often difficult to perform if the practitioner has small hands, especially if the client has large legs. Another variation makes performance of this test easier. The client's knee is supported in slight flexion by placing a pillow or bolster under the knee. The practitioner is then more easily able to get her inferior hand underneath the proximal tibia in order to pull it in an anterior direction.

SUGGESTIONS FOR TREATMENT: The proper course of treatment for an ACL injury is determined by a number of different factors. If the injury is not severe, conservative forms of treatment using braces and therapeutic exercise are often the treatment of choice. If the injury is quite severe or the client is involved in activities (like competitive athletics) which will be limited because of the diminished function of the ACL, surgery may be indicated. An active rehabilitation program will be required in order to gain the most benefit of the surgical procedures. Massage is not a treatment that is indicated for direct effect on ACL injuries because the ligament lies within the joint and is inaccessible to the practitioner's fingers. However, massage applications can greatly enhance relief of secondary muscle spasm and biomechanical alterations which usually accompany ligament sprain. Improvements in mobility and success in the postsurgical rehabilitation program can be aided by the effective application of certain massage approaches.

---

(31) CONDITION:
POSTERIOR CRUCIATE LIGAMENT SPRAIN

Figure 5-8a
Posterior view of the knee showing a tear to the posterior cruciate ligament

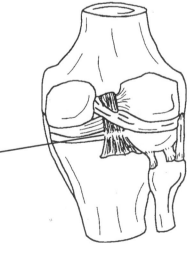

CHARACTERISTICS: The posterior cruciate ligament (PCL) is responsible for preventing posterior movement of the tibia in relation to the femur. In that respect its action is just opposite that of the ACL. It also provides some resistance to rotary stress on the knee joint. It is most resistant to lateral rotation of the tibia in relation to the femur. However, the PCL is most often injured as it is resisting posterior movement of the tibia. We are often injured when we encounter a strong force in the opposite direction of our forward movement. A direct blow on the anterior portion of the tibia, especially near its proximal end, would force it to move in a posterior direction in relation to the femur. This movement will stress the PCL. This can happen when a person falls and hits an object on the ground with the anterior tibia as they fall. Another common mechanism of injury is for a passenger in the front seat of a car to hit the anterior tibia on the dashboard as they are thrown forward in an accident.

ASSESSMENT: As with the ACL injury there are several different ways to test for the presence of a PCL disruption. The mechanism of injury will tell a great deal about which primary ligament structure is injured. The client may hear an audible "pop" associated with the injury and is likely to feel pain deep within the joint. It is also likely that there will be a sense of instability in the knee as if it may "give way". Laxity or tearing in the PCL can be further clarified with the posterior drawer test.

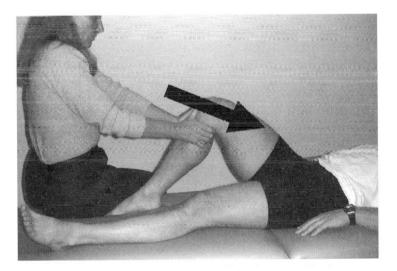

Figure 5-8b
*Posterior drawer test
for injury to the posterior
cruciate ligament.*

POSTERIOR DRAWER TEST- The client is in a supine position with the knee flexed and the plantar surface of the foot flat on the table. The therapist may anchor the client's foot by sitting on the end of the forefoot. The therapist will grasp the proximal end of the tibia with both hands and place her thumbs on the tibial tuberosity. The therapist will push the tibia in a posterior direction (indicated by the arrow). If there is movement or a "mushy" end-feel it is indicative of damage to the PCL.

SUGGESTIONS FOR TREATMENT: Treatment for PCL injuries will be very similar to that for ACL injuries. See the description above on ACL injuries for specifics.

(32) CONDITION: MEDIAL COLLATERAL LIGAMENT SPRAIN

valgus force

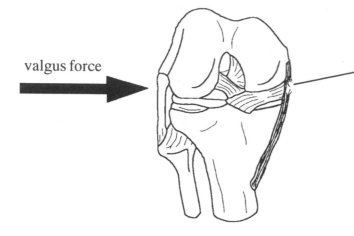

Figure 5-9a
Anterior view of the right knee with the patella removed showing tearing of the medial (tibial) collateral ligament

CHARACTERISTICS: The medial collateral ligament (MCL), which is also sometimes called the tibial collateral ligament, is designed to prevent excessive valgus stress to the knee. A valgus stress is one that is directed in a medial direction from the lateral side of the knee. This ligament is part of the "Terrible Triad" mentioned in the section on ACL sprains. It is frequently injured in combination with the ACL and the medial meniscus. The most common mechanism of injury is a direct blow to the outside of the knee. This often happens in contact sports when one player hits another player on the lateral side of the knee, especially with the weight of the body behind the blow. The player who is being hit is usually weight bearing on the leg that is hit and so the knee is forced to buckle inwards.

ASSESSMENT: The person will usually feel sharp pain immediately on the medial side of the knee and may hear an audible "pop". Pain may subside to a minimal level shortly after the injury. This is because primary nerve fibers to the area have been disrupted as well. Determination of a sprain to the MCL is done by use of the Valgus Stress Test.

Figure 5-9b
Valgus stress test for injury to the medial collateral ligament.

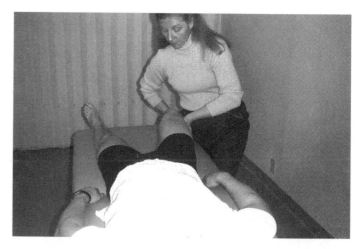

VALGUS STRESS TEST- The client is in a supine position on the treatment table. The therapist will place the superior hand on the lateral joint line so that the middle of the palm of the hand is right over the joint line. The inferior hand will be used to offer a stabilizing (resisting) force to the movement of the upper hand. The client's knee can be tested in full extension and slight flexion (about 20° to 30°). The practitioner will stabilize the leg with the inferior hand and place a straight valgus force to the lateral side of the knee with the superior hand. No movement should be sensed in a ligament with good integrity. If the ligament is damaged, a slight "mushy" or soft end-feel may be present. Visual gapping on the medial side of the knee joint may also be present.

SUGGESTIONS FOR TREATMENT: As with all other ligament sprains in the knee, the nature of treatment may vary quite a bit depending on the severity of the ligament damage. Severe or grade 3 ligament sprains often require surgical intervention. Mild or moderate sprains will often be treated using more conservative measures such as protective braces to offer additional support while the ligament heals. Because the MCL is a superficial knee ligament, massage applications can play an important role in rehabilitation of MCL sprains. Once the initial phase of injury has subsided, deep friction applications may be helpful in preventing excess scar tissue buildup around the injury site. This approach will also help keep the ligament from scarring down to adjacent soft tissue and bony structures as it goes through its fibrous rebuilding phase. Significant muscular spasm may be present with MCL injuries and general applications to the thigh and leg muscles will also be indicated to help reestablish proper biomechanical balance around the joint.

---

(33) CONDITION: LATERAL COLLATERAL LIGAMENT SPRAIN

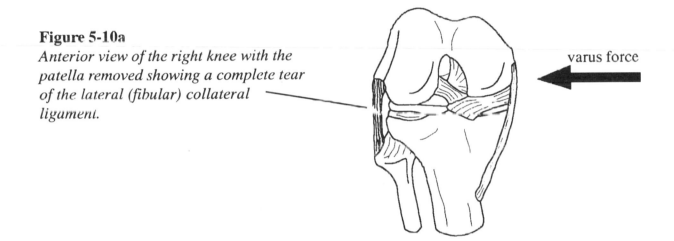

Figure 5-10a
Anterior view of the right knee with the patella removed showing a complete tear of the lateral (fibular) collateral ligament.

varus force

CHARACTERISTICS: The lateral collateral ligament (LCL) sprain is far less common than the MCL sprain. The LCL, also called the fibular collateral ligament, is responsible for preventing excessive varus stress to the knee. A varus stress is one directed in a lateral direction from the medial side of the knee. One reason LCL injuries are less frequent is that the opposite leg will usually protect the knee from varus forces. If it is injured, there will frequently be injury to other structures such as the cruciate ligaments or the iliotibial band.

ASSESSMENT: The client will report something in the history that involves a varus stress to the knee or some motion of the knee which has given the LCL acute tensile stress. There is likely to be immediate pain on the lateral side of the knee. As with the other ligament injuries to the knee, pain may not be present after the immediate onset of the injury. Clarification of injury to the LCL is determined by use of the Varus Stress Test.

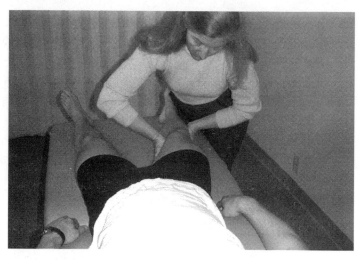

Figure 5-10b
Varus stress test for injury to the lateral collateral ligament.

VARUS STRESS TEST- This test is very similar in its application to the valgus stress test. The client is in a supine position and the practitioner will have the superior hand on the medial side of the knee joint. The palm will be right over the joint line. The inferior hand will be used to provide a valgus (stabilizing) force to the leg. The knee can be tested in both full extension and slight flexion (about 20° to 30°). The practitioner will apply a varus force (laterally directed force from the medial side) to the medial joint line of the knee. If there is a soft or "mushy" end-feel to the movement or visible joint gapping, the LCL may be deficient. The amount of movement will vary depending on the severity of the ligament injury.

SUGGESTIONS FOR TREATMENT: As with the MCL, treatment for LCL injuries will vary with the severity. Grade 3 sprains will usually warrant surgery, whereas grade 1 and 2 sprains will often be treated through conservative measures such as bracing and modification of activity. The LCL is also a superficial ligament and is therefore accessible for massage treatment. Deep friction approaches may be helpful in forming a functional scar once the initial acute phase of the injury has subsided. As with the MCL, these friction approaches are helpful to reduce adhesion between the ligament and adjacent soft-tissues and bone. General massage applications to the thigh and leg are also likely to be helpful in reestablishing proper biomechanical balance. The muscles surrounding the knee will often go into a protective spasm immediately following an injury to the ligaments of the knee.

---

(34) CONDITION: MENISCAL INJURY

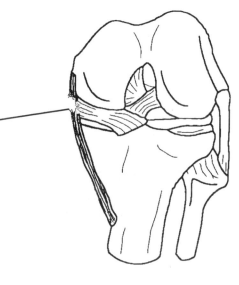

Figure 5-11a
Anterior view of the left knee with the patella removed. The medial meniscus is damaged in conjunction with the medial collateral ligament. Fibers of the medial collateral ligament attach to the meniscus causing it to be injured also.

CHARACTERISTICS: The lateral and medial menisci are cartilage "disks" that are in the knee joint between the tibia and femur. Their primary role is shock absorption and maintaining a proper gliding contact surface for the femoral condyles on the tibial plateau. Excessive compressive or rotational forces or severe traction forces on the knee may cause damage to the meniscus. The meniscus will usually tear, but it may be damaged in a way such that a loose fragment of the meniscal cartilage is floating in the joint. Meniscal injuries are often hard to detect because there is no nerve supply on the inner two thirds of the meniscus so there may not be any pain associated with the meniscal injury.

ASSESSMENT: Assessment of meniscal injuries is difficult because of the lack of vascularity and nerve supply. There are several different tests used to determine the presence of meniscal injuries. The Apley compression and distraction tests may be used to help clarify ligamentous versus meniscal involvement in the injury.

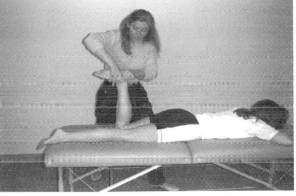

Figure 5-11b
The Apley compression test for meniscal damage

APLEY COMPRESSION TEST- This test is used to identify the presence of a tear or disruption to the meniscus. The client is in a prone position with the knee of the involved side flexed to approximately 90°. The practitioner will place stress directly down on the tibia and then gently rotate the tibia medially and laterally. If pain or discomfort arises from that motion, it is likely that there is meniscal involvement. However, the rotary movement may also cause pain to injured ligamentous structures. This can be clarified by use of the Apley distraction test.

Figure 5-11c
The Apley distraction test for meniscal damage

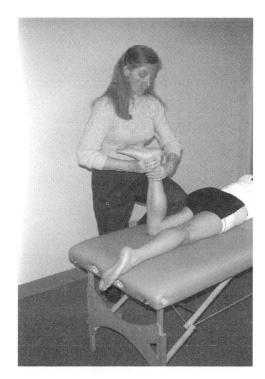

APLEY DISTRACTION TEST- The same starting position is used for the distraction test as for the compression test. The client is in a prone position with the knee flexed to 90°. The practitioner will stabilize the femur to the treatment table by placing her knee on the back side of the client's thigh to hold it to the table. The practitioner will then lift up on the foot putting a pulling (distraction) force on the tibia. Once the distraction force is applied, the practitioner will then medially and laterally rotate the tibia. The distraction force takes stress off the meniscus. If pain is still felt with this movement, there is a good indication that the injured structure may be ligamentous.

SUGGESTIONS FOR TREATMENT: Meniscal injuries are usually treated with surgery. The meniscus may be repaired, the injured tissue may be removed, or the whole meniscus may be removed. Meniscus transplants are currently being practiced for some severe conditions as well. Massage applications may play a role in the rehabilitation of a meniscus injury, but will have little effect in correcting the primary problem. The massage applications used during the rehabilitation phase will be geared toward improvement of biomechanical balance and reduction of fibrous scar tissue that may result from prolonged immobilization and lack of appropriate movement.

(35) CONDITION: PATELLOFEMORAL PAIN SYNDROME

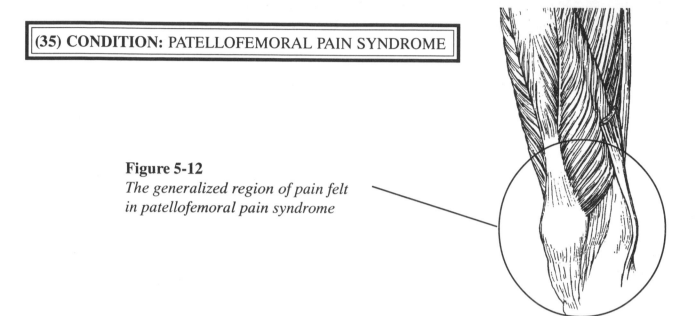

Figure 5-12
The generalized region of pain felt in patellofemoral pain syndrome

CHARACTERISTICS: Patellofemoral Pain Syndrome (PFPS) is similar to shin splints in that it has become a catchall term for anterior knee pain that is felt under the patella. There is no specific set of symptoms and no one particular tissue which is involved. This condition may also go by the names of patellofemoral compression syndrome, patellar malalignment syndrome, or lateral patellar compression syndrome. There are several common symptoms and predisposing factors which are present.

PFPS is a condition of chronic onset anterior knee pain. This pain will often feel like it is under the patella. The client will often have a positive movie sign (see the special terms and concepts section). This condition is frequently caused by problems such as patellar tracking disorders which may eventually lead to other degenerative changes like chondromalacia patella. Weakness of the VMO will often lead to an increase in lateral patellar tracking which may cause the anterior knee pain frequently described as PFPS. Clients may also complain of knee pain associated with activities such as jumping or climbing stairs which use quadriceps strength predominantly.

ASSESSMENT: Since there is not a set condition or specific dysfunction that is termed PFPS, assessment of this condition may be quite variable. It will mostly be derived from information obtained in the history. Important factors are anterior knee pain that appears to be the result of a chronic onset, a large Q angle, problems with correct patellar tracking, and/or a weak VMO. A large Q angle, greater than 15^0 in men or 20^0 in women, may be involved. The increase in the Q angle causes the patella to have a greater likelihood of deviating laterally during normal quadriceps activity. These factors may be all or part of the problem with PFPS. However, since it is not a clearly defined condition, it is difficult to say exactly what the primary causative factors are.

SUGGESTIONS FOR TREATMENT: PFPS is frequently treated with conservative measures. This will include bracing or supports that attempt to improve patellar tracking, modification of activity, stretching and strength training. It will be wise for the client to avoid activities that use a great deal of quadriceps strength such as climbing, squatting, or jumping. Stretching of the quadriceps and hamstring muscle groups will be helpful as will a general strengthening program for the quadriceps. It will be most important to strengthen the vastus medialis muscle. However it is very difficult to isolate this muscle when doing strengthening exercises. Massage applications are likely to be effective when applied to the quadriceps muscle group, especially the vastus lateralis and the lateral retinaculum. If excess tension can be relieved on the vastus lateralis and the lateral retinaculum, this can improve patellar tracking.

(36) CONDITION: CHONDROMALACIA PATELLA

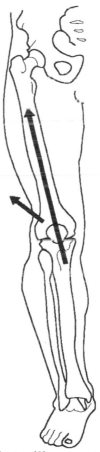

Figure 5-13a
Lateral patellar tracking. One of the primary causes of chondromalacia patella. The large arrow represents the general angle of pull of the quadriceps muscle group. The small arrow indicates the tendency this force has to pull the patella in a lateral direction. The pull in a lateral direction will drag the patella over the femoral condyles, damaging the cartilage underneath the patella.

CHARACTERISTICS: Chondromalacia is a gradual onset condition that will present with anterior knee pain that is felt under that patella. It is created by compression and degeneration of the articular cartilage on the underside of the patella. This will happen as a result of improper patellar tracking or certain bony configurations such as overly large femoral condyles. The patella needs to track straight in the groove between the femoral condyles, and if it does not, it will cause excess friction and wear on the cartilage on the underside of the patella. Clients who have chondromalacia will frequently report the same types of signs and symptoms as with PFPS, however, they may often be more pronounced.

ASSESSMENT: The client will usually report chronic anterior knee pain. They will be likely to have a positive movie sign and have knee pain when ascending or descending stairs. The presence of chondromalacia can be confirmed through arthroscopic surgery. However, its presence is highly likely if the client has pain during a patellofemoral compression test or has a positive Clarke's sign.

Figure 5-13b
The patellofemoral compression test for the presence of chondromalacia.

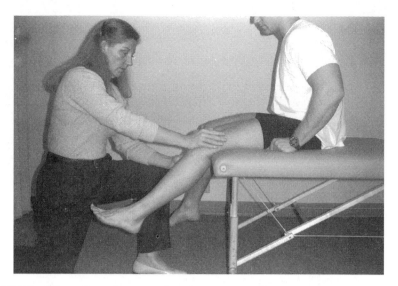

PATELLOFEMORAL COMPRESSION TEST- The client is seated on the edge of the treatment table. The therapist places a hand directly over the client's patella and places a moderate amount of compression on the patella. The client is then instructed to extend the knee while the therapist continually applies the compression. If pain is felt under the patella during this movement, it is likely that there is some softening and degeneration of the cartilage.

Figure 5-13c
Clarke's sign testing for chondromalacia

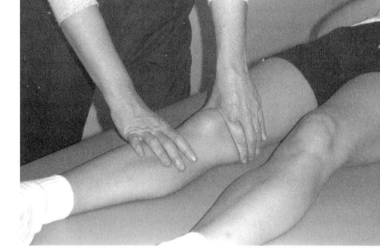

CLARKE'S SIGN- The client is in a supine position on the treatment table with the knee extended. The upper portion of the patella will be stabilized by the webbing between the thumb and the hand. The practitioner will press down (posterior direction) on the distal thigh in order to firmly stabilize the position of the patella. The client will then be asked to contract the quadriceps muscle while the practitioner holds pressure on the superior portion of the patella. IMPORTANT NOTE: This test can be quite painful for the client even if they are barely symptomatic. You may want to have them begin the quadriceps contraction slowly. If they say any effort causes discomfort, that should be considered as a positive test. It does not take a great deal of effort or pressure on the practitioner's part because almost anyone will feel pain with this test if enough pressure is exerted.

SUGGESTIONS FOR TREATMENT: Chondromalacia is most often treated with modifications of activity, rest, and strengthening of the quadriceps muscles. Attempts to correct any patellar tracking disorders just like those that were mentioned in the section on PFPS are also helpful. Massage applications may be helpful in reducing improper patellofemoral biomechanics that are the result of an overly tight vastus lateralis or lateral patellar retinaculum. Massage is also helpful in restoring tension balances between the quadriceps and hamstring muscle groups especially when combined with specific stretching techniques.

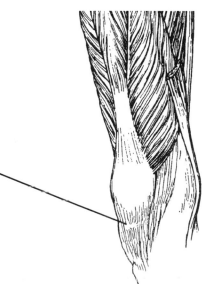

---

(37) CONDITION: PATELLAR TENDINITIS

Figure 5-14
Microtearing of tendon fibers of infrapatellar tendon - patellar tendinitis.

CHARACTERISTICS: Patellar tendinitis is also frequently called "jumper's knee" because of the common occurrence in people who do a great deal of jumping such as basketball players. This is a gradual onset condition that involves irritation and inflammation of the infra-patellar tendon (sometimes called the patellar ligament because of its attachment to both the patella and the tibia). The client will most often complain of pain associated with activity that decreases with rest. The pain during activity may come on and then subside with increasing levels of movement. Pain will be felt in the region just below (inferior) to the patella, especially with pressure. Sometimes clients will report that this pain feels like it goes into the knee joint. As with other tendinitis conditions the problem is excessive or improper repetitive use of the quadriceps muscles.

ASSESSMENT: The presence of patellar tendinitis is best determined by information in the history that indicates overuse combined with certain signs that will be evident in the physical examination. The infra-patellar tendon will be tender to pressure and resisted knee extension. It is important to note that because of the mechanical role of the quadriceps, pain may not be elicited with a manual resistive test, though the client will feel it during certain active motions such as squatting. The tension generated during a manual resistive test may not match the normal force requirements of the quadriceps muscle group. In discriminating patellar tendinitis from other anterior knee pain conditions such as chondromalacia, pay particular attention to the tenderness of the infrapatellar tendon. The infrapatellar tendon should not be painful if only chondromalacia is present.

SUGGESTIONS FOR TREATMENT: Patellar tendinitis is most often treated with various conservative measures. This may include modification of activities to alleviate those that involve running, jumping, or squatting. In addition, ice applications following any strenuous activity will help decrease the inflammatory response in the tendons. Strength training programs for the quadriceps are also used to help build their resistance to fatigue. However, this should be done in a careful manner so as not to increase the level of irritation to the patellar tendon. Deep transverse friction massage applications are quite effective in helping to realign fibrous scar tissue and create mobility in the tendon fibers. Any deep friction applications should be combined with appropriate treatment of the quadriceps muscle group in order to reduce overall tension.

(38) CONDITION: OSGOOD-SCHLATTER'S DISEASE

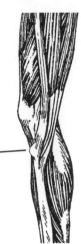

Figure 5-15
*Osgood-Schlatter's disease.
Enlarged tibial tuberosity created by
tensile stress on the apophysis.*

CHARACTERISTICS: The term disease is somewhat of a misnomer for this condition. Most people think of a disease as some type of organic or cellular dysfunction. This is an overuse condition that primarily affects adolescents and boys more often than girls. It is characterized by an inflammatory reaction of the distal attachment of the quadriceps tendon at the tibial tuberosity. It happens more in adolescents because of changes in bone growth and size will make this area more susceptible to overuse stress. There will be pain and inflammation at the distal portion of the patellar tendon and the tibial tuberosity will be tender. If it has progressed significantly, there will be a pronounced bump on the tibial tuberosity which will make it large. It was originally thought to be an avulsion of the tibial tuberosity, but now it is believed to be an inflammatory reaction.

PES ANSERINE — TIBIAL TUBEROSITY

ASSESSMENT: Presence of Osgood-Schlatter's Disease is determined by a history involving frequent use or overuse of the quadriceps muscle group. Age is a factor as this condition is much more frequent in adolescents. Tenderness to palpation is likely to be present at the tibial tuberosity. An enlarged tibial tuberosity is also an indicator.

SUGGESTIONS FOR TREATMENT: Treatment for this condition will focus on relieving excessive stress on the attachment point of the quadriceps group. This is usually done through strength and flexibility programs for both the quadriceps and the hamstrings. It is important to remember that optimum muscle function, and therefore decreases in muscle tension, can best be achieved when there is a strength/flexibility balance. Therefore strength training should be combined with flexibility training or vice/versa. Massage applications to the quadriceps to decrease general tension in this muscle group may also be effective.

(39) CONDITION: PREPATELLAR BURSITIS

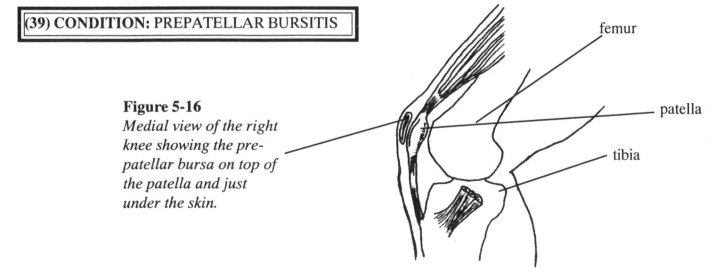

Figure 5-16
*Medial view of the right
knee showing the pre-
patellar bursa on top of
the patella and just
under the skin.*

femur

patella

tibia

CHARACTERISTICS: The prepatellar bursa is located just under the skin directly on top of the patella. This bursa can become inflamed or irritated from a single direct trauma such as a blow to the anterior knee, or it may become irritated from repetitive compression stress such as kneeling on the knees. The pain will most often be felt above the patella and there may be local redness and swelling accompanying this condition. The client will frequently complain of pain in the region as the knee is flexed because the skin over the bursa becomes increasingly tightened as the knee is flexed.

ASSESSMENT: Prepatellar bursitis is most easily assessed by a few simple signs and symptoms. There will be swelling and redness superficial to the patella. This area may be tender to a moderately light touch. Resisted motions of the knee will not cause additional discomfort and the pain will be limited to the area just above (anterior) to the patella.

SUGGESTIONS FOR TREATMENT: As with many other bursitis conditions, prepatellar bursitis will respond best to rest and modification of activity. If this condition has come on gradually from repeated compression such as frequent kneeling, it will be best to refrain from that activity. Ice applications may be helpful to avoid painful swelling. If the swelling is severe, the region may be aspirated (the withdrawing of fluid by a syringe). Massage applications will not be of much help with this condition and in fact, if applied to the area would likely be detrimental.

---

(40) CONDITION: ILIOTIBIAL BAND FRICTION SYNDROME

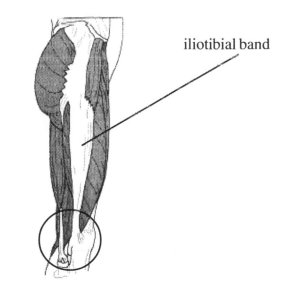

iliotibial band

Figure 5-17a
Iliotibial band friction syndrome.
The circled area indicates the pri-
mary area where pain is felt.

CHARACTERISTICS: Although iliotibial band (ITB) friction syndrome involves the thigh and hip, the prominent area of pain is felt on the lateral side of the knee. The iliotibial band courses over the lateral side of the femoral epicondyle. Excessive tensile stress on the iliotibial band will create friction between the band and the femoral epicondyle as it crosses over. The friction may be caused by several different factors. Tightness in the muscles on the superior end of the ITB such as the gluteus maximus or the tensor fasciae latae may create greater tensile stress on the band. Running on sloped surfaces will also put greater tensile stress on the leg on the "downhill" side. Enlarged femoral epicondyles or any type of lateral protrusion from the femoral epicondyle is also likely to increase the friction. The friction may also be increased by a genu varum alignment. The friction causes irritation of the iliotibial band fibers. There is also a bursa underneath the iliotibial band which can get irritated as a result of compression. Clients will usually feel pain with activity that will subside with rest. The pain will be felt on the lateral side of the femur and in severe cases may be recreated with passive or active flexion and extension of the knee. The pain or discomfort will often be worse when going up or down stairs.

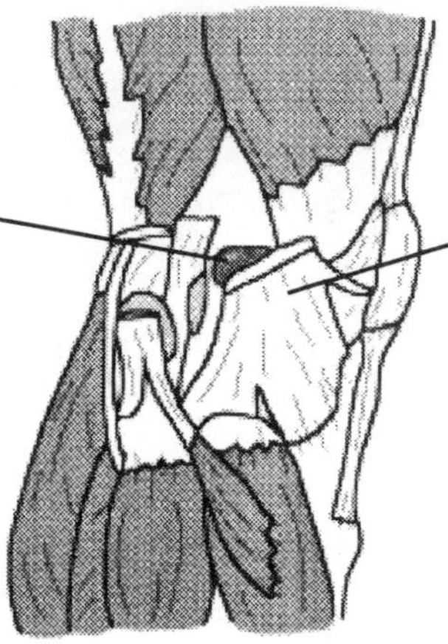

Figure 5-17b
Lateral view of the knee showing the bursa just beneath the distal portion of the iliotibial band.

distal attachment of the iliotibial band

ASSESSMENT: The client will have something in the history that indicates overuse of the flexion/extension motion at the knee. Pain will be felt at the lateral region of the knee, and it will usually subside with rest. Pain may be created with active or passive range of motion tests. There may be some tenderness over the lateral joint line of the knee. Tightness of the ITB is a significant factor in this condition. The Ober test can be used to determine if the iliotibial band is excessively tight.

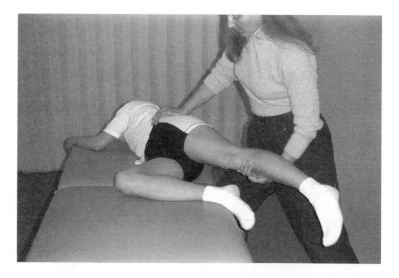

Figure 5-17c
The Ober test for tightness in the iliotibial band

OBER TEST- The client is in a side-lying position on the treatment table with the affected leg being the uppermost. The unaffected knee will be flexed to help provide stability. The client may also be encouraged to hold on to the edge of the treatment table for stability. The therapist will bring the affected limb into abduction and then into about 20^0 of (hyper)extension. Once the limb has reached this position the therapist will slowly lower the limb. If the limb stays at a level of horizontal or above, it is indicative of tightness in the iliotibial band. If the limb naturally descends to horizontal or angles downward the client is considered not to have iliotibial band tightness.

Although the Ober Test will demonstrate excessive tightness in the ITB, ITB friction may often happen in the absence of visible tightness with the Ober Test. Another way to test for it is with the Noble compression test.

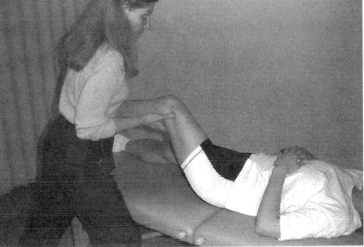

Figure 5-17d
Noble compression test examining for the presence of iliotibial band friction syndrome

NOBLE COMPRESSION TEST - The client is in a supine position. The hip is flexed and the knee is flexed to approximately 90^0. The practitioner will place her thumb on the ITB just slightly proximal to the femoral epicondyles. Pressure is exerted on the ITB by the thumb while the practitioner uses the other hand to passively extend and flex the knee. If ITB friction syndrome is present the client will likely feel pain at about 30^0 of flexion. This pain will be the same sensation of discomfort that is felt during activity or when the condition is aggravated.

SUGGESTIONS FOR TREATMENT: ITB friction syndrome will often be treated with modification of activity and a stretching program to decrease the tensile stress on the ITB by decreasing tension in the muscles on its proximal end. Ice applications may be helpful in decreasing any inflammatory reaction around the knee. Massage applications are likely to be very helpful. Treatment should focus on the gluteal muscles and the tensor fasciae latae in order to reduce tension on the ITB. Massage to the quadriceps and hamstrings will also be important. Deep friction massage techniques to the distal portion of the ITB may help prevent fibrous scar tissue buildup in the region. However, if the irritation is caused by chronic compression of the bursa underneath the distal portion of the ITB, deep friction over this area may make the condition worse. These massage techniques should be followed up with effective stretching and movement of the area in order to enhance mobilization. Stretching can be accomplished by using the same position as the Ober Test.

---

(41) CONDITION: MUSCLE STRAIN

CHARACTERISTICS: Acute overloading of musculotendinous structures in the thigh and knee region will lead to muscle strains. The muscles acting on the knee, such as the quadriceps and hamstrings, are capable of generating large amounts of force. Muscle strains to these muscles can be frequent and severe. The adductor muscles of the inner thigh are also quite susceptible to muscle strain. The mechanical design of some of these muscles makes them particularly susceptible to strain. The hamstrings, for example, cross two joints and therefore have to be able to generate force over those two joint segments. They are opposed by the quadriceps muscle group which is much stronger and acts across only one joint (except for the rectus femoris). This is one factor that increases the frequency of hamstring strains. The nature of movement also dictates that these large muscles of the thigh are often exposed to high eccentric forces. Eccentric overloading is the leading cause of muscle strain.

ASSESSMENT: Knowledge of anatomy will be crucial in determining the presence of muscle strains. These conditions may have a number of symptoms depending on their severity. See the section in the beginning of the book on muscle strains for a more complete description of the differences between the various grades of strain. Determination of muscle pain or weakness may be based on the use of various manual resistive tests which isolate that muscle. Manual resistive tests for the single plane movements of the knee were included at the beginning of this chapter.

SUGGESTIONS FOR TREATMENT: Any discussion of the treatment of muscle strains must be considered relative to the degree of the strain. For instance, the method of treatment for a grade 1 strain will be different from that of a severe grade 3 strain. In most instances, muscle strains will be treated with rest from the offending activity, some type of anti-inflammatory treatment, stretching in the post-acute phase, and gradual strengthening as the injury repair progresses. Massage applications such as deep transverse friction are quite effective in helping to create a functional scar that is strong, yet pliable enough not to impair the proper use of the tissue. Massage is also very helpful during the rehabilitative phase to decrease muscle spasm which may have occurred immediately after the injury and is preventing the proper biomechanical balance from returning.

(42) CONDITION: NEUROMUSCULAR PAIN

CHARACTERISTICS: Any muscle in the body is capable of holding an increased level of neurological activity and maintaining a spasm. The spasm of that muscle will then lead to increased pain and disturbed biomechanical function. Muscle spasm can be perpetuated by various stimuli including chemicals like caffeine, certain medications, myofascial trigger points, or emotional stress. Muscle spasm of the thigh muscles acting on the knee often happens as a secondary result of other injury such as ligament sprains. The pain may be relieved by rest, but simple activities of daily living will often cause the pain to resurface. Because of the role of these muscles in locomotion, it is difficult to fully rest them and give them the optimum conditions for returning to normal function.

ASSESSMENT: The muscles will frequently be painful in certain areas to palpation, may demonstrate a decreased range of motion, and may be somewhat painful to resisted isometric contraction or stretching. They may contain painful myofascial trigger points which refer pain or other autonomic phenomena to remote areas. Familiarity with common trigger point pain referral patterns will aid in the determination of which muscles may be involved. See the sections above for references on manual resistive tests and range of motion testing for selected muscles of the thigh and knee region.

SUGGESTIONS FOR TREATMENT: These conditions respond very favorably to massage applications. Since muscular spasm is a primary component of these conditions, a technique like massage that is highly effective in addressing muscular spasm is very effective in reducing the complaint. If the condition arises from poor postural or biomechanical function, movement reeducation is very helpful, and in most cases necessary, as an adjunctive treatment. Because of the large size of the muscles in this area and the relative mobility of the lower extremity, massage applications that use active and passive motion during the massage techniques will help get good results with these types of conditions.

Quick Reference for Conditions of the Knee and Thigh

REGION OF PAIN	ONSET	POSSIBLE CAUSE	REF.
INTERIOR OF KNEE JOINT	ACUTE	ACL SPRAIN	30
INTERIOR OF KNEE JOINT	ACUTE	PCL SPRAIN	31
MEDIAL KNEE JOINT	ACUTE	MCL SPRAIN	32
LATERAL KNEE JOINT	ACUTE	LCL SPRAIN	33
MEDIAL OR LATERAL KNEE JOINT LINE	ACUTE OR CHRONIC	MENISCAL INJURY	34
ANTERIOR KNEE	CHRONIC	PATELLOFEMORAL PAIN SYNDROME	35
KNEE UNDERNEATH PATELLA	CHRONIC	CHONDROMALACIA PATELLA	36
ANTERIOR KNEE	CHRONIC	PATELLAR TENDINITIS	37
ANTERIOR PROXIMAL TIBIA	CHRONIC	OSGOOD-SCHLATTER'S DISEASE	38
SUPERFICIAL ANTERIOR KNEE	ACUTE OR CHRONIC	PRE-PATELLAR BURSITIS	39
LATERAL KNEE	CHRONIC	ILIOTIBIAL BAND FRICTION SYNDROME	40
ANY MUSCLE	ACUTE OR CHRONIC	MUSCLE STRAIN	41
ANY MUSCLE	CHRONIC	NEUROMUSCULAR PAIN	42

CHAPTER 6

HIP AND PELVIS CONDITIONS

Overview of Common Single Plane Movements of the Hip and Pelvis

Active and passive ROM tests and manual resistive tests will require a knowledge of basic joint mechanics and functional anatomy for the regions surrounding the joint. The practitioner must know what constitutes normal, pain free motion in order to determine if there is a problem. The discussions of active ROM tests, passive ROM tests, and manual resistive tests will utilize the terms listed below. Familiarity with these terms and how they apply to the body will be essential in order to gain valid information from the assessment. All joint angle measurements which are included are measured from the neutral position, which is anatomical position. In order to properly understand and simplify joint mechanics, the movements at the joints described below have been broken down into single plane movements. That means movement in one of the three primary planes of motion - sagittal, frontal, or transverse. Although this greatly simplifies the analysis of movement, it should be kept in mind that this classification rarely happens in actual human movement. Almost every movement we make will be a combination of movements in different planes. However, muscle or joint dysfunction can often be accurately pinpointed by comparing certain single plane movements. The primary muscles involved with each action are listed under the description of that action. Note that this may not include every muscle which is involved in that action, only the primary ones.

Flexion- The anterior region of the thigh is brought up toward the chest. Movement occurs in the sagittal plane. Average range of motion in hip flexion is dependent on the position of the knee. If the knee is extended average range of motion is approximately 90^0. If the knee is flexed average hip flexion will reach 120^0 or greater. The primary muscles involved in hip flexion are:

Psoas
Iliacus
Rectus Femoris
Sartorius

Extension- in anatomical position the hip is in full extension. Extension is also the movement returning to anatomical position from any flexed position. When the movement goes past anatomical position in the direction of extension it is called hyperextension. Average range of motion in extension is about 20^0. The primary muscles involved with extension are:

Biceps Femoris
Semimembranosus
Semitendinosus
Gluteus Maximus

Medial/Internal Rotation- This movement is best visualized if the knee is brought into 90^0 of flexion. This makes the movement of the hip easier to see. From anatomical position with the knee flexed the hip will rotate medially as the foot moves in a lateral direction. Average range of motion in medial rotation of the hip is 30^0. The primary muscles involved in medial rotation are:

> **Adductor Longus**
> **Adductor Brevis**
> **Adductor Magnus**
> **Gluteus Medius**
> **Gluteus Minimus**

Lateral/External Rotation- As with the medial rotation, this movement is best visualized with the knee flexed. As the hip rotates laterally the foot will move in a medial direction. Average range of motion in lateral rotation is approximately 60^0. The primary muscles involved in lateral rotation are:

> **Piriformis**
> **Obturator Internus**
> **Obturator Externus**
> **Quadratus Femoris**
> **Gemellus Superior**
> **Gemellus Inferior**

Abduction- The thigh and leg move away from the midline of the body while moving in the frontal plane. It is quite difficult to abduct only one limb at a time. When one abducts, there is a corresponding abduction that occurs in the other limb. Average range of motion in abduction for each limb is considered to be about 45^0. Therefore it may appear as if it is relatively easy to achieve 90^0 of abduction with one limb. What is actually occurring is that the pelvis is moving on the stationary limb and creating 45^0 of movement at each hip joint. The primary muscles involved in abduction are:

> **Tensor Fasciae Latae**
> **Gluteus Minimus**
> **Gluteus Medius**
> **Gluteus Maximus**
> **Sartorius**

Adduction- The hip is in adduction in anatomical position. Adduction is also the movement that brings the hip back into anatomical position from some degree of abduction. The hip is not able to move past its normal anatomical position in adduction without making adjustments because it will contact the opposite leg. If the hip is either slightly flexed or slightly hyperextended, or if the opposite limb is flexed or hyper extended to get it out of the way, the hip can move into about 30^0 of adduction. The primary muscles involved in adduction are:

> **Adductor Longus**
> **Adductor Brevis**
> **Adductor Magnus**
> **Pectineus**
> **Gracilis**

Active Range of Motion Tests

Active range of motion tests for the hip will include the six single plane movements described above. It may be easiest to perform them in a standing position.

Passive Range of Motion Tests

These tests are sometimes difficult to perform because of the weight of the lower limb and positioning factors. The therapist may have to use some originality in determining how to place the client in the most effective position to get an accurate determination of passive movement potential. It may be necessary to change positions for each movement that is being tested. The nature of end-feel at the hip joint will be an important indicator of healthy or pathological tissues.

The end-feel for flexion depends on the position of the knee. If the knee is extended, the end-feel will be tissue stretch as the hamstring muscles reach their limit of elongation. If the knee is flexed, the end-feel may be tissue stretch with the hamstrings again if the client is not very flexible. If the client is flexible, however, the end-feel will be more like soft-tissue approximation as the quadriceps encounter the torso.

The end-feel for extension is a "ligamentous" tissue stretch. This tends to be more abrupt than a muscle tendon tissue stretch. The iliofemoral ligament will limit extension going past 20^0. Note that in some people it may appear that (hyper)extension can go past 20^0. However, this movement is created by the pelvis tilting anteriorly.

The end-feel for medial rotation is tissue stretch. It is the lateral rotators of the hip which limit this movement.

The end-feel for lateral rotation is tissue stretch. It is created by the medial rotators and adductors.

The end-feel for abduction is tissue stretch. Abduction is limited by the stretching of the adductor muscles. If an individual is very flexible the end-feel may be bone-to-bone as the femoral neck presses against the acetabulum.

The end-feel for adduction is soft-tissue approximation if the opposite limb is in anatomical position or tissue stretch if the adducting limb is allowed to move further into adduction.

Manual Resistive Tests

The next section includes illustrations and descriptions of manual resistive tests for the six single plane movements of the hip joint. Remember that each of these movements can be performed in either of the two ways described earlier to perform manual resistive tests.

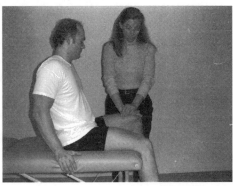

Figure 6-1
Resisted flexion of the hip.

The client is in a seated position on the edge of the treatment table. By having the client seated, the hip is already close to its neutral position for testing flexion. The client will attempt to flex the hip, lifting it off the table and the therapist will offer resistance.

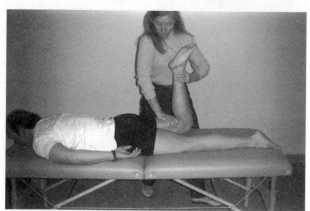

Figure 6-2
Resisted extension of the hip

The client is in a prone position on the table. The hip is brought into a slight degree of hyperextension. The client will attempt to hyper extend further and the therapist will offer resistance with the hand which is placed on the posterior thigh. The knee is flexed so that the effort of the hamstrings will be focused on extending the hip and not attempting to flex the knee.

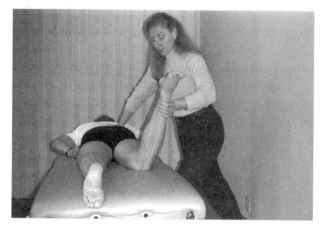

Figure 6-3
Resisted internal rotation of the hip

The client is in a prone position on the treatment table. The knee is flexed to 90°. The therapist will bring the client's hip into partial medial rotation. The client will attempt to medially rotate the hip further and the therapist will offer resistance. This is an example of the situation that works easier if the therapist puts the limb in the test position and tells the client to hold it there while the therapist attempts to move it in the opposite direction. The movement of medial rotation of the hip is hard to describe to the client and is a movement with which they are probably unfamiliar. It is therefore easier just to have them hold a position.

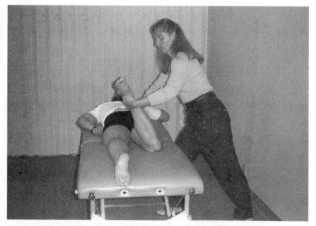

Figure 6-4
Resisted external rotation of the hip.

The client is in a prone position on the treatment table. The hip is brought into a partial lateral rotation position. The therapist will have the client attempt to further rotate the hip laterally while offering resistance. As with the medial rotation, this movement is easier to perform if the therapist instructs the client to hold the position while resistance is offered in the opposite direction of the desired movement.

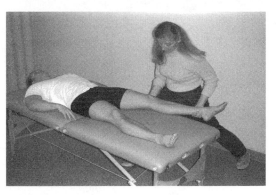

Figure 6-5
Resisted abduction
of the hip

The client is in a supine position on the treatment table. The limb is brought into partial abduction. The therapist places one hand above the knee and one hand below the knee. Both hands are on the outside of the lower extremity. The client is instructed to abduct the hip further while the therapist offers resistance. The therapist should primarily offer resistance with the hand that is above the knee joint.

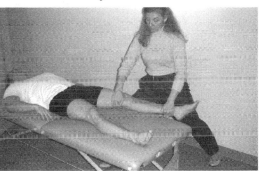

Figure 6-6
Resisted adduction
of the hip.

This client is supine on the treatment table. The limb is brought into a slight degree of abduction. The therapist will place one hand above the knee and one hand below the knee. Both hands are on the inside of the lower extremity. The client is instructed to further adduct the limb while the therapist offers resistance. Again, as in the test of abduction, the resistance should be primarily offered by the therapist's hand which is above the knee.

GUIDE TO CONDITIONS OF AND SPECIAL REGIONAL ORTHOPEDIC TESTS OF THE HIP AND PELVIS

Structural and Postural Deviations

(43) CONDITION: ANTERIOR PELVIC TILT

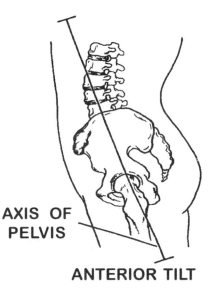

AXIS OF PELVIS

ANTERIOR TILT

Figure 6-7a
Anterior tilt of the pelvis
(Illustration courtesy of
Educational Graphics)

CHARACTERISTICS: A proper balance of the pelvis relies on numerous factors such as tightness in low back muscles, leg length, or tightness in hip or lower extremity muscles. One of the most common structural problems of the pelvis is an anterior tilt. Anterior tilt of the pelvis also will increase the natural lordosis in the spine and aggravate low back problems. The increase in pelvic tilt will also functionally lengthen the hamstring muscles. This may cause the hamstring muscles to be more prone to tensile stress injuries.

ASSESSMENT: Anterior pelvic tilt is most appropriately assessed from a lateral view. Anterior pelvic tilt will increase the lordosis in the low back and make the buttocks more prominent. It may cause the upper torso to lean back in an attempt to offset the forward lean of the torso caused by the pelvis tilting the lumbar vertebrae forward. Anterior pelvic tilt may be caused by tightness in the iliopsoas muscle. A special test for investigating iliopsoas tightness is a modification of the Thomas test.

Figure 6-7b
Thomas test for
tightness of iliopsoas muscle.

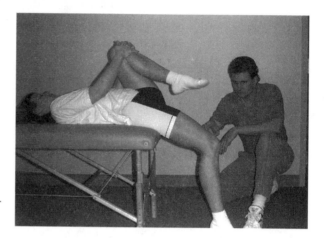

THOMAS TEST- The client is instructed to back up to the edge of the treatment table and just barely rest the buttocks on the table. The client will then grasp the knee of the side opposite to the one that is being examined. The therapist will help the client roll back onto her back while maintaining the hip of the non-test side in about 135^0 of flexion. Once in this position, the therapist will examine the position of the thigh on the test side (in this picture it is the right side). If the thigh is at horizontal or above, there may be tightness present in the iliopsoas. If the thigh is below horizontal, the iliopsoas is at least normal length and maybe more. When the thigh is parallel to the ground, the knee should be in about 90^0 of flexion. If the knee has less than 90^0 of flexion, this indicates that the rectus femoris may be tight. Note that, as in Figure 6-7b, if the thigh drops below horizontal, and the knee is in less than 90^0 of flexion, that doesn't necessarily mean the rectus femoris is tight. If the thigh were brought back up to horizontal, the knee would hang at about 90^0.

SUGGESTIONS FOR TREATMENT: Since this problem often is created by imbalance in the soft-tissues, it is a structural condition ideally suited for treatment with massage. However, the practitioner must take a comprehensive look at all the factors which may be involved in creating the condition. The abdominal muscles may be weak and functionally lengthened. They will likely need to be strengthened. The lumbar spinal extensors, especially the erector spinae, will often be tight. The iliopsoas is often a prime creator of anterior pelvic tilt by pulling the lumbar vertebrae forward. Decreasing tension in it will be very helpful. The rectus femoris may also be tight and contributing to the anterior tilt. A strength imbalance between the quadriceps and hamstrings in which the hamstrings are weakened from being functionally lengthened may also contribute to the problem. Strengthening the hamstrings would then be indicated.

(44) CONDITION: POSTERIOR PELVIC TILT

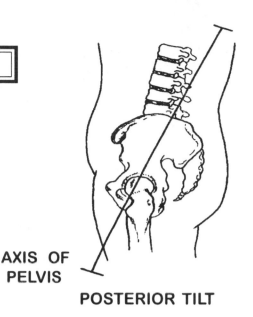

Figure 6-8
*Posterior tilt of
the pelvis.*
*(Illustration courtesy of
Educational Graphics)*

**AXIS OF
PELVIS**

POSTERIOR TILT

CHARACTERISTICS: This is the opposite of anterior pelvic tilt. In this condition the lumbar lordosis is decreased so that the low back region appears almost flat. This gives a "tucking under" effect to the pelvis. The intervertebral disks were designed for a certain amount of lordosis and this lordosis is necessary for shock absorption. If the lumbar region loses its lordosis, as it does during posterior pelvic tilt, there is likely to be increased compression on the lumbar vertebrae and their disks.

ASSESSMENT: As with the anterior tilt, this condition is best assessed from a lateral view. The pelvis appears to be rotating in a posterior direction. As the pelvis tilts posteriorly the buttocks become less prominent and the low back will flatten out to become almost straight. There is often a corresponding rounding of the shoulders that appears with posterior tilt of the pelvis. Tight hamstrings may also be a causative factor.

SUGGESTIONS FOR TREATMENT: As with the anterior pelvic tilt, this may be primarily a soft-tissue problem. There is likely to be shortening and tightening in the abdominal muscles and hamstrings. A functional lengthening and weakening may also be present in the lumbar spinal extensors, the iliopsoas, and the rectus femoris. In addition to massage applications that are directed at loosening the tight muscles, strengthening of the hip flexors and spinal extensors would be indicated.

(45) CONDITION: LATERAL PELVIC TILT

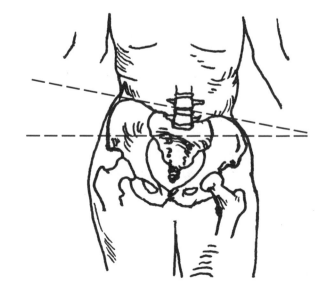

Figure 6-9
*Lateral tilt of
the pelvis.*

99

CHARACTERISTICS: In addition to tilting forward or backward the pelvis may also be inclined to one side more than the other. This may happen for a number of different reasons. Tightness in the lumbar lateral flexors, such as the quadratus lumborum, on one side may pull the pelvis more to one side than the other. There may be a structural or functional leg length difference. Understanding the difference between a structural (true) leg length discrepancy and a functional leg length discrepancy is important.

Tightness in the lateral flexors of the lumbar spine may pull the pelvis into a lateral tilt. This lateral tilt may make one leg appear shorter than the other. Some health care practitioners will look at the legs in a supine or prone position and declare that a leg length difference is present simply from visual inspection. However, there are too many variables which may be present that can alter the apparent difference in leg length. In physical examination a good estimate of leg length can be derived by taking a tape measure and measuring the limb from the greater trochanter of the femur to the medial malleolus. A more accurate way is to measure the length of the bones on an X-Ray film. If one bone is longer than the other, this is a structural or "true" leg length discrepancy. If not, then the apparent leg length discrepancy is considered to be a functional discrepancy. A functional discrepancy means that for the purposes of normal function, one leg is acting as if it is shorter than the other.

ASSESSMENT: Lateral pelvic tilt is best assessed from the front or back. Place a hand or finger on the ASIS of each side of the pelvis. Look at the level compared to the other side. They should be in the same horizontal plane with each other. If there is a significant lateral tilt of the pelvis, it is likely to create a functional scoliosis as well. This means that the spine may be curving in a lateral direction. Yet it is a structural problem of muscle tightness that is causing the scoliosis as opposed to a congenital factor.

SUGGESTIONS FOR TREATMENT: It is likely that the lateral tilt of the pelvis is caused by muscular imbalance that will respond well to massage approaches. Massage and stretching should be addressed to the lumbar muscles on the "high" side. In addition to addressing the lateral flexors, the therapist should attempt to achieve an ideal muscular balance around the whole hip and pelvis region by addressing all the muscles involved in the six primary single plane movements of the hip.

Common Injury Conditions

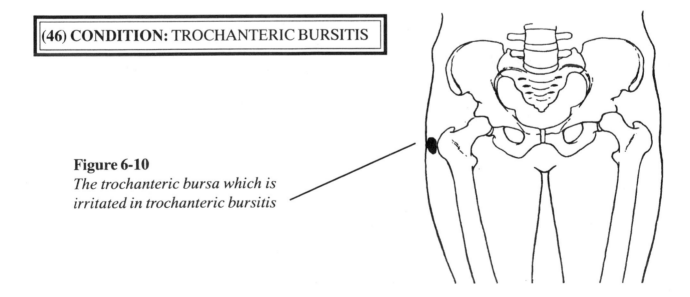

(46) CONDITION: TROCHANTERIC BURSITIS

Figure 6-10
The trochanteric bursa which is irritated in trochanteric bursitis

100

CHARACTERISTICS: There is a bursa which lies over the greater trochanter of the femur and under the iliotibial band. If this bursa is aggravated from either repetitive compression or by a direct blow, it is likely to become inflamed and cause pain and discomfort directly over the greater trochanter of the femur. Activities which involve repetitive flexion/extension movements of the hip, such as cycling, are frequent causes. Also because there is not a great deal of soft-tissue over the greater trochanter, it is subject to the bursitis condition from direct blows that might happen during a fall on the hip, for example.

ASSESSMENT: The client is likely to have factors in the history which would indicate the presence of either direct trauma to the lateral hip region or some activity that would be likely to cause a great deal of friction to the trochanteric bursa. Tightness in the iliotibial band may be a contributing factor as the iliotibial band rubs over the trochanter. A client with trochanteric bursitis will have pain directly over the greater trochanter of the femur and may report difficulty sleeping or lying on his/her side. Inflammation may be present directly over the greater trochanter, but it is often difficult to tell because of the amount of adipose or muscle tissue which may be in the area.

SUGGESTIONS FOR TREATMENT: As with many bursitis conditions, the best method of treating this is with rest and modification of any offending activity. An inflamed bursa will generally subside if the irritating forces which caused it to become inflamed are removed. If the condition is caused by overuse, then massage applications to the gluteal muscles, abductors, flexors, and extensors would be indicated. It is often tightness in these muscles which will cause increased tension on the iliotibial band causing it to rub harder over the greater trochanter. It may be a good idea to see if the client has a tight iliotibial band to start with. This can be done by using the Ober Test (see reference #40).

(47) CONDITION: SACROILIAC (S-I) JOINT DYSFUNCTION

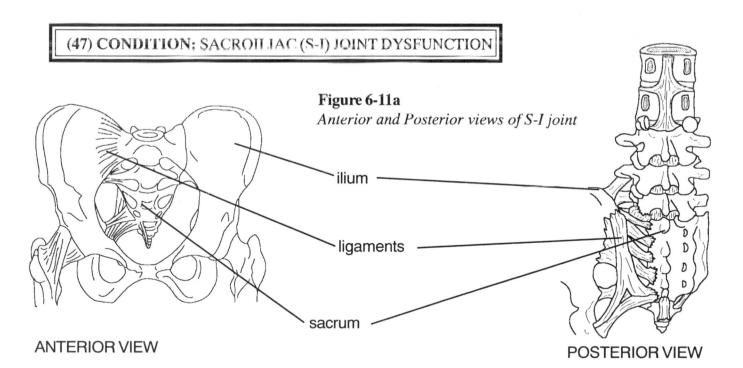

Figure 6-11a
Anterior and Posterior views of S-I joint

ilium

ligaments

sacrum

ANTERIOR VIEW   POSTERIOR VIEW

CHARACTERISTICS: The S-I joint has a unique structural design. The sacrum distributes the weight of the upper body across the two halves of the pelvis so that the bone acts primarily as a wedge. The S-I joint is considered relatively immobile but certain forces may disrupt the proper mechanical function of the joint. Chronic postural stresses or acute injuries may stretch or weaken the ligament structures which hold the joint intact. This will then lead to irritation of the articular surfaces of the joints.

101

NO TIGHTEN

ASSESSMENT: The client is likely to report pain in the low back or sacral region. The pain may be associated with particular movements or sitting for long periods. Pain may also be referred to the gluteal region or down the posterior portion of the leg. Dysfunction of the sacroiliac ligaments can be tested with the gapping test or the FABER test.

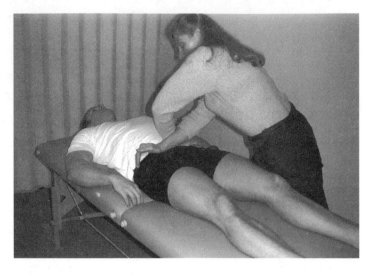

Figure 6-11b
Gapping test for
S-I joint dysfunction

GAPPING TEST - The client is in a supine position on the treatment table. The therapist will place on hand over each ASIS of the client. Because of the direction of the force that is to be applied, the therapist may find it easier to cross the arms to the opposite ASIS as is depicted in the picture. The therapist then puts pressure in a downward and lateral direction on each ASIS. This downward and lateral pressure will stress the sacroiliac ligaments and the sacroiliac joint. If pain is caused in the S-I joint, gluteal region, or down the posterior leg, it is an indicator that S-I joint pathology may be involved.

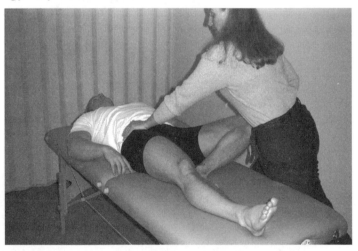

Figure 6-11c
FABER test for
S-I joint dysfunction.

FABER TEST- This test may go by several different names. It is also called Patrick's test or the figure 4 test (named for the position of the legs during the test). The client is in a supine position. One leg is straight out and the other leg is in the FABER position. FABER is an acronym that stands for Flexion ABduction and External Rotation. If the client is unable to place the foot on the opposite leg, the foot may be placed against the medial side of the straight leg. The therapist will use one hand (on the ASIS) to stabilize the pelvis and the opposite hand to apply a slight bit of pressure downward on the flexed knee. A client with S-I joint dysfunction is likely to feel discomfort in the S-I region as a result of this test.

SUGGESTIONS FOR TREATMENT: The most appropriate form of treatment for S-I joint dysfunction will rely on what is the primary causative factor. There are a number of things that may be leading to the S-I irritation. Stretching and mobilization of the S-I joint is likely to be helpful. Massage approaches to the muscles acting on the pelvic girdle will also be helpful to normalize biomechanical balance around the pelvis.

(48) CONDITION: HIP POINTER

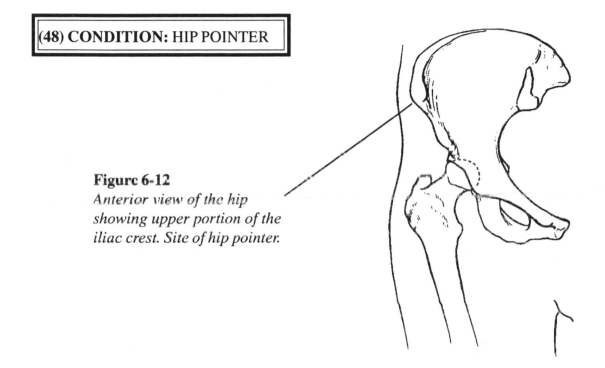

Figure 6-12
Anterior view of the hip showing upper portion of the iliac crest. Site of hip pointer.

CHARACTERISTICS: A hip pointer is a general term that is used differently by different practitioners. It most often refers to a contusion or direct trauma to the iliac crest. This happens frequently in contact sports or in situations in which a person falls directly on a hard surface. The term hip pointer is also used in certain circles to refer to avulsion conditions of the oblique muscles that tear away from the iliac crest. These are usually the result of a sudden lateral flexion of the torso against resistance.

ASSESSMENT: A history of a sudden blow or direct trauma to the upper iliac crest region will be characteristic. There may be point tenderness over the area and some swelling may be present. If the client attempts to laterally flex the torso to the opposite side, it is likely to increase the pain.

SUGGESTIONS FOR TREATMENT: A hip pointer is best treated in the manner of most acute injuries - with rest, and some type of anti-inflammatory treatment. Ice is effective because it may also decrease neurological activity that will allow early mobilization to be effective. Massage applications will not be indicated until the post-acute phase of the injury (several days). At that time, attention can be given to the oblique muscles, lumbar lateral flexors and abductors of the hip to help alleviate any muscle spasm which has developed secondary to the injury.

(49) CONDITION: PIRIFORMIS SYNDROME

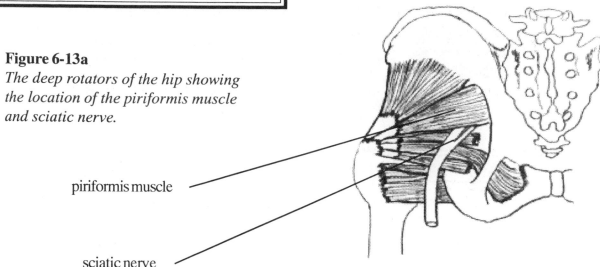

Figure 6-13a
The deep rotators of the hip showing the location of the piriformis muscle and sciatic nerve.

piriformis muscle

sciatic nerve

CHARACTERISTICS: Piriformis syndrome is a nerve compression syndrome that will mimic the symptoms of a lumbar disk protrusion on a spinal nerve. The piriformis muscle is a primary lateral rotator of the hip. The sciatic nerve goes over the other five deep hip rotators and under the piriformis as it is leaving the sacral plexus and descending the limb as depicted in Figure 6-13a. In some instances the sciatic nerve will come over the top of the piriformis muscle or actually perforate the muscle. This is much more likely to lead to problems with the sciatic nerve being compressed. Depending on its severity, pain may be felt in the immediate gluteal region, down the posterior thigh, or all the way down the leg if the compression on the nerve is severe.

ASSESSMENT: The client is most likely to report pain in the gluteal region or pain that goes down the posterior portion of the thigh. The pain may be aggravated by prolonged sitting or activities that use the hip muscles extensively. Stretching the piriformis muscle is likely to increase the pressure on the sciatic nerve if the muscle is compressing the nerve. If this increases pain, it is likely that there is piriformis involvement. This can be done with the piriformis test.

Figure 6-13b
Piriformis test examining for impingement of the sciatic nerve by the piriformis muscle.

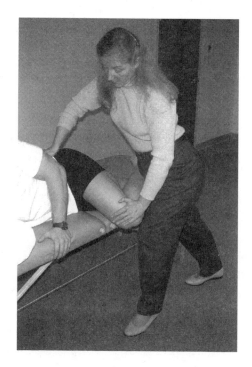

PIRIFORMIS TEST- The client is in a side-lying position with the hip and knee of the affected side flexed. It is helpful if the client is at the edge of the table so that there is room for the test leg to drop off the table. The client will bring the hip into medial rotation and the therapist will use one hand to stabilize the pelvis and the other hand to apply a gentle amount of pressure downward on the knee to help stretch the piriformis further. The therapist must watch to make sure that the pelvis stays close to vertical, and that the client doesn't attempt to twist the torso in order to accomplish the movement.

SUGGESTIONS FOR TREATMENT: If the primary problem is resulting from piriformis tightness, massage applications and stretching aimed at the gluteal muscles and deep rotators of the hip will be helpful. The therapist must be careful when applying pressure in the gluteal region to make sure that the pressure does not contact the irritated sciatic nerve and make the discomfort worse. Since the pain from this condition is originating from a nerve compression, it is of no benefit to continue applying pressure on a painful nerve.

(50) CONDITION: MUSCLE STRAIN

CHARACTERISTICS: Acute overloading of musculotendinous structures in the hip and pelvis will lead to muscle strains. However, except for the adductors of the thigh, muscle strains in this region are not very *NO* common. When they do occur the forces necessary to create them are usually quite large.

ASSESSMENT: Knowledge of anatomy will be crucial in determining the presence of muscle strains. These conditions may have a number of symptoms depending on their severity. See the section in the beginning of the book on muscle strains for a more complete description of the differences between the various grades of strain. Determination of muscle pain or weakness may be based on the use of various manual resistive tests which isolate that muscle. Manual resistive tests for the six single plane movements of the hip and pelvis were included at the beginning of this chapter.

SUGGESTIONS FOR TREATMENT: Any discussion of the treatment of muscle strains must be considered relative to the degree of the strain. For instance, the method of treatment for a grade 1 strain will be quite different from that of a severe grade 3 strain. In most instances muscle strains will be treated with rest from the offending activity, some type of anti-inflammatory treatment, stretching in the post-acute phase, and gradual strengthening as the injury repair progresses. Massage applications such as deep transverse friction are quite effective in helping to create a functional scar that is strong, yet pliable enough not to impair the proper use of the tissue. Massage is also very helpful during the rehabilitative phase to decrease muscle spasm which may have occurred immediately after the injury and is preventing the proper biomechanical balance from returning.

(51) CONDITION: NEUROMUSCULAR PAIN

CHARACTERISTICS: Any muscle in the body is capable of holding an increased level of neurological activity and maintaining a spasm. The spasm of that muscle will then lead to increased pain and disturbed biomechanical function. Muscle spasm can be perpetuated by various stimuli including chemicals like caffeine, certain medications, myofascial trigger points, or emotional stress. The pain may be relieved by rest, but simple activities of daily living will often cause the pain to resurface. These conditions are some of the most frequent problems encountered by any health care practitioner who works with the musculoskeletal system.

ASSESSMENT: The muscles will frequently be painful in certain areas to palpation, may demonstrate a decreased range of motion, and may be somewhat painful on a resisted isometric contraction. They may contain painful myofascial trigger points which refer pain or other autonomic phenomena to remote areas. Chronic overuse, postural or biomechanical imbalances which are evident through the history may be indicating factors. See the sections above for references on manual resistive tests and range of motion testing for selected muscles of the hip and pelvis.

SUGGESTIONS FOR TREATMENT: These conditions respond very favorably to massage applications. Since muscular spasm is a primary component of these conditions, a technique like massage that is effective in addressing muscular spasm is very helpful in reducing the complaint. If the condition arises from poor postural or biomechanical function, movement reeducation is very helpful, and in most cases necessary, as an adjunctive treatment.

Quick Reference for Conditions of the Hip and Pelvis

REGION OF PAIN	ONSET	POSSIBLE CAUSE	REF.
LATERAL HIP	ACUTE OR CHRONIC	TROCHANTERIC BURSITIS	46
LOWER LUMBAR, SACROILIAC REGION	ACUTE OR CHRONIC	SACROILIAC JOINT DYSFUNCTION	47
ILIAC CREST	ACUTE	HIP POINTER	48
GLUTEAL REGION OR POSTERIOR LOWER EXTREMITY	CHRONIC	PIRIFORMIS SYNDROME	49
ANY MUSCLE	ACUTE OR CHRONIC	MUSCLE STRAIN	50
ANY MUSCLE	CHRONIC	NEUROMUSCULAR PAIN	51

CHAPTER 7

LUMBAR AND THORACIC SPINE CONDITIONS

SPECIAL TERMS AND CONCEPTS

1) ANNULUS FIBROSIS- is the portion of the fibrocartilage intervertebral disk that surrounds the more gel-like center known as the nucleus pulposus. The annulus is like the concentric rings in the cross sectional view of a tree. Fibers are arranged in an oblique fashion in order to give the annulus the ability to withstand multidirectional stress.

2) FACET- is the articulating surface between adjacent vertebra. The superior facet of one vertebra articulates with the inferior facet of the one above it. The contact surface at the facet joint is rather small, yet, it is the only place where adjacent vertebra articulate directly with each other.

3) NUCLEUS PULPOSUS- is the gel-like substance in the center of an intervertebral disk that acts like a hydraulic cushion. It is the nucleus pulposus which protrudes from the center of the disk when a disk is herniated or ruptured.

4) IPSILATERAL- is a term meaning to the same side. It is used in the description of rotation movements of the spine. For example, an ipsilateral rotator muscle is one that rotates the body to the same side - the muscle on the right side of the body rotates the body to the right.

5) CONTRALATERAL- means to the opposite side. In describing rotation movements of the spine it refers to the movements that go to the opposite side from where the muscle is located. For example a contralateral rotator muscle on the right side of the body will rotate the body to the left.

Overview of Common Single Plane Movements of the Lumbar and Thoracic Spine

Active and passive ROM tests and manual resistive tests will require a knowledge of basic joint mechanics and functional anatomy for the regions surrounding the joint. The practitioner must know what constitutes normal, pain free motion in order to determine if there is a problem. The discussions of active ROM tests, passive ROM tests, and manual resistive tests will utilize the terms listed below. Familiarity with these terms and how they apply to the body will be essential in order to gain valid information from the assessment. All joint angle measurements which are included are measured from the neutral position, which is anatomical position. In order to properly understand and simplify joint mechanics, the movements at the joints described in each regional section below have been broken down into single plane movements. That means movement in one of the three primary planes of motion - sagittal, frontal, or transverse. Although this greatly simplifies the analysis of movement it should be kept in mind that this classification rarely happens in actual human movement. Almost every movement we make will be a combination of movements in different planes. However, muscle or joint dysfunction can often be accurately pinpointed by comparing certain single plane movements. The primary muscles involved with each action are listed under the description of that action. Note that this may not include every muscle which is involved in that action, but only the primary ones. It should be noted that movements of the spine differ from movements of many other areas of the body in that movement is not occurring in one particular joint in most cases. The movements created in the spine are happening as a result of small degrees of movement between each of the individual vertebral segments. The average range of motion figures given for the spine should not be taken as rigid standard because there are many different joints that contribute to the range of motion that is listed. Use these figures as a general guide.

Flexion- a movement which brings the torso down toward the anterior portion of the thighs. Flexion of the thoracolumbar region happens primarily in the lumbar vertebra. Average range of motion in flexion is 40^0 to 60^0. Muscles involved in flexion include:

> **Psoas (Major & Minor)**
> **Rectus Abdominus**
> **External Oblique**
> **Internal Oblique**
> **Transverse Abdominus**

Extension- a movement of the spine which returns the body to anatomical position from a flexed position. If the movement in that direction continues past upright, it is called hyperextension. This is the movement commonly associated with the exercise called "back bends". Average range of motion for extension is 20^0 to 35^0. The primary muscles involved in extension are:

> **Erector Spinae**
> **Semispinalis**
> **Multifidus**
> **Quadratus Lumborum**

Lateral Flexion- a movement in the frontal plane in which the torso bends to the side. Pure lateral flexion does not have any flexion or extension of the torso happening with it. However, in normal movement these motions will often be combined together. Average range of motion in lateral flexion is 15^0 to 20^0. The primary muscles involved with lateral flexion are:

> **Latissimus Dorsi**
> **Erector Spinae**
> **Quadratus Lumborum**
> **Transversospinalis**
> **External Oblique**
> **Intertransversarii**

Rotation- a movement in which the torso is turned to the right or left. Since it is the central axis of the body that is turning, rotation is labeled right or left instead of medial or lateral. Rotation happens primarily in the thoracic region. Rotation may only be about 10^0 to 15^0 in the lumbar spine, but is about 45^0 in the thoracic spine. The primary muscles involved with rotation are:

Semispinalis
Multifidus
Rotatores

Active Range of Motion Tests

Active range of motion tests for the lumbar and thoracic spine will include the four single plane movements described above. The movements of lateral flexion and rotation should be performed to each side. It may be easiest to perform them in a standing position.

Passive Range of Motion Tests

These tests are sometimes difficult to perform because of the weight of the torso and positioning factors. The therapist may have to use some originality in determining how to place the client in the most effective position to get an accurate determination of passive movement potential. A sitting position may be the best option. The end-feel for all the movements of the spine when there is no dysfunction is tissue stretch.

Manual Resistive Tests

The next section includes illustrations and descriptions of manual resistive tests for the four single plane movements of the thoraco-lumbar spine. Remember that each of these movements can be performed in either of the two ways described earlier to perform manual resistive tests.

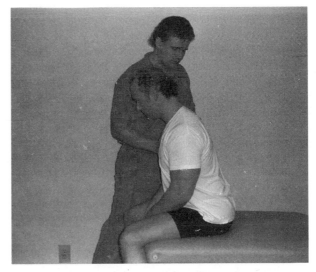

Figure 7-1
Resisted flexion of the torso

The client is in a seated position on the edge of the treatment table. The therapist is slightly to the side and front of the client with one hand on the client's upper chest region. The therapist may place the other hand on the client's back just for stability. The therapist will have the client attempt to bend the torso forward while offering resistance.

111

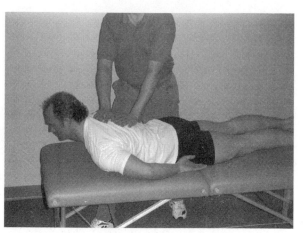

Figure 7-2
*Resisted extension
of the lumbar spine.*

The client is prone on the treatment table. The therapist will place a hand on the upper back region. The client is instructed to attempt to raise the torso off the table while the therapist offers a slight bit of resistance. In many instances the weight of the body will be enough to engage the muscles significantly so that added resistance is not needed.

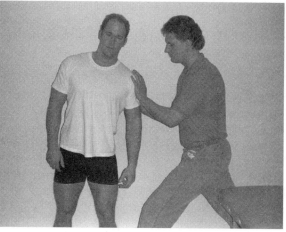

Figure 7-3
*Resisted lateral flexion
of the torso*

The client is in a standing position. The therapist is at the client's side with both hands on the client's shoulder. The client brings the torso into a small degree of lateral flexion. The therapist will tell the client to hold this position while trying to push the client back into the upright position.

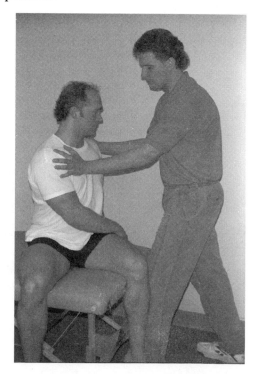

Figure 7-4
*Resisted rotation of
the torso*

The client is seated on the edge of the treatment table. In order to anchor the pelvis to keep it stationary it may be helpful to have the client straddle the corner of the treatment table as shown in the picture. The therapist will place one hand on each of the client's shoulders. The client is brought into a partial rotation position and asked to hold that position as the therapist attempts to turn the client's torso back to the front.

Structural and Postural Deviations

NOTE ON SPINAL CONDITIONS: The nature of pathological conditions in the spine is unique. It is often difficult to determine exactly what the problem is because there can be so many variable factors to consider. What may be the ideal exercise or treatment for one person may make another person feel worse even though their symptoms may have been identical to start with. When working with conditions of the spine it is always advisable to consult with other practitioners (physicians, chiropractors, physical therapists, etc.) who have special expertise in working with a variety of spine conditions. However, some practitioners will place less emphasis on the role of soft-tissue involvement with spine conditions. You will have to determine each practitioner's philosophy about spine problems to see if that model is consistent with what you find.

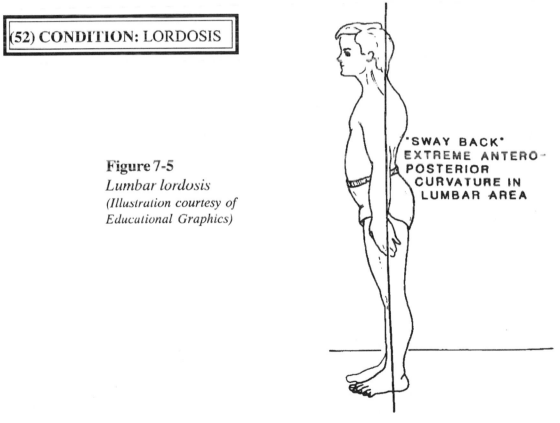

(52) CONDITION: LORDOSIS

"SWAY BACK"
EXTREME ANTERO-
POSTERIOR
CURVATURE IN
LUMBAR AREA

Figure 7-5
Lumbar lordosis
(Illustration courtesy of
Educational Graphics)

LORDOSIS

CHARACTERISTICS: Lordosis was mentioned in the chapter on hip and pelvis conditions as being associated with anterior pelvic tilt. The natural curvature of the lumbar spine, which is convex in an anterior direction (bending toward the front), is considered the normal lumbar lordosis. If it becomes excessive, however, it is considered a pathological condition. An increased lumbar lordosis is often seen in conjunction with anterior pelvic tilt, a tight iliopsoas muscle, tight lumbar spinal extensors, and a variety of other soft tissue compensations. There are a number of factors which may lead to an exaggerated lumbar lordosis, such as sitting in poor posture all day or wearing high-heel shoes for long periods.

ASSESSMENT: As with the anterior pelvic tilt, this condition is best assessed from a lateral position. Look for exaggerated curvature in the lumbar spine, prominence of the gluteal region, and a backward leaning upper torso. It may also be helpful to examine the client in a supine position with the legs extended out in front of them. In a normal lumbar lordosis there is just enough room to slide one hand snugly under the low back. If the lordosis is exaggerated there will be more room to slide the hand under the lumbar region. See the description for the Thomas test (reference # 43) for evaluation of iliopsoas tightness also.

SUGGESTIONS FOR TREATMENT: Treatment options will vary greatly with what is the primary cause of the lumbar lordosis. Some things that may be helpful include massage and stretching to the lumbar spinal extensor muscles. Changes in body mechanics for daily activities will often be necessary for making a lasting change. Some practitioners will also advocate strengthening of the abdominals.

---

(53) CONDITION: KYPHOSIS

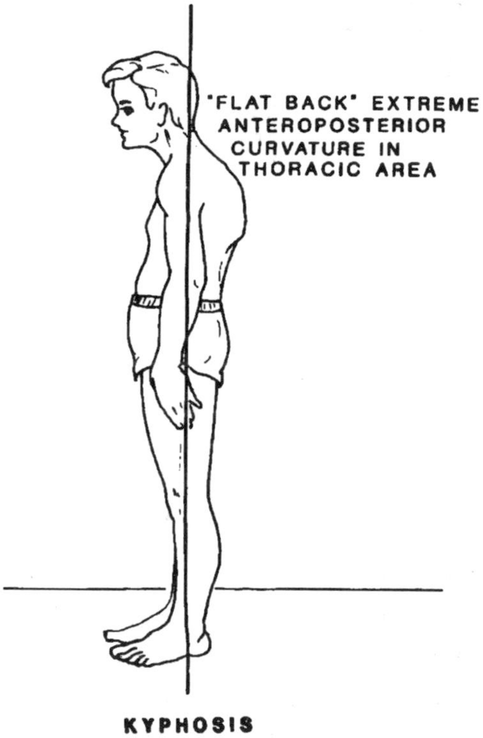

Figure 7-6
Thoracic kyphosis
*(Illustration courtesy of
Educational Graphics)*

"FLAT BACK" EXTREME
ANTEROPOSTERIOR
CURVATURE IN
THORACIC AREA

KYPHOSIS

CHARACTERISTICS: Kyphosis is a curvature of the upper thoracic region which is convex in a posterior direction. It is often associated with poor postural alignment of the neck and shoulders. It is usually developed over a long period of time. There may be a number of factors which bring in on. It is often seen in people who are quite tall as they make an effort to communicate and interact with those around them who are much shorter. This condition involves chronic strain on the upper thoracic and neck muscles as they attempt to defy gravity in holding up the upper torso and neck. In a normal alignment the weight of the upper torso and head would be evenly distributed throughout the skeletal structure.

ASSESSMENT: This condition is easy to identify. Examine the client from a lateral direction. If you have a grid wall or some vertical reference like a plumb line it is even better. Look for the head and upper back to be ahead of the gravity bearing line through the center of the body. There will be curvature to the upper thoracic region that is convex in a posterior direction.

SUGGESTIONS FOR TREATMENT: In many instances kyphosis has been such a slowly developing long-term postural problem that it takes a great deal of time to reverse the process. Massage applications and stretching to the anterior shoulder and chest musculature will be helpful. Attention should also be addressed to the posterior cervical muscles. Movement and postural reeducation will be necessary in order to make lasting changes.

(54) CONDITION: SCOLIOSIS

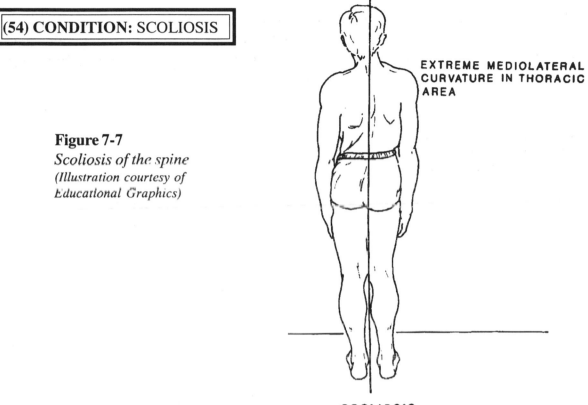

EXTREME MEDIOLATERAL CURVATURE IN THORACIC AREA

Figure 7-7
Scoliosis of the spine
(Illustration courtesy of Educational Graphics)

SCOLIOSIS

CHARACTERISTICS: Scoliosis is a lateral curvature of the spine. It is often congenital, in which case many therapeutic interventions have limited effectiveness. In other cases it is a functional scoliosis, or one that has developed in reaction to various other postural distortions such as unequal leg length (see reference # 45 for a discussion of leg length). Scoliosis is likely to lead to a host of other soft-tissue problems because of the muscle and fascial shortening that is involved. Lumbar disk protrusions may become more common because of the unequal distribution of weight forces on the lumbar vertebra.

ASSESSMENT: Depending on the severity of the scoliosis it may be hard to detect. If it is severe, the torso will be deviating to one side when viewed from behind. It may be helpful to palpate and note the position of each spinous process and see if they are in a straight line or do they deviate from the vertical. Looking at the inclination of the shoulders may be helpful as well. When a scoliosis is present the shoulders have to compensate and adjust to the movement in order to bring the head back to vertical. This will also cause an imbalance of the shoulder muscles.

SUGGESTIONS FOR TREATMENT: There are numerous theories about how to treat scoliosis. It will be most important to determine what has caused the scoliosis in the first place. If it is severe and congenital, it may be treated surgically by placing rods directly adjacent to the spine in order to hold the spine straight. In other conditions when it is not as severe, massage applications may be helpful to normalize the muscle balance around the spine. Most of the attention should be put on the muscles on the "short" side of the curvature.

Common Injury Conditions

(55) CONDITION: LUMBAR DISK PATHOLOGY

Figure 7-8a
Tearing and ruture of an intervertebral disk
(Illustration courtesy of Educational Graphics)

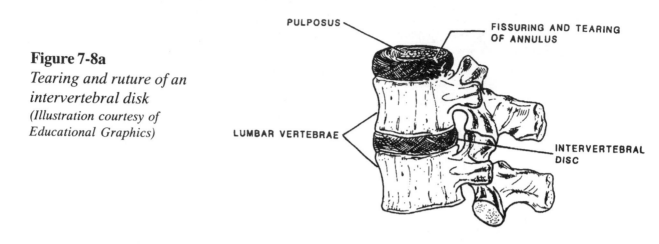

LATERAL VIEW

CHARACTERISTICS: There are a number of problems that may occur to the lumbar disks, most of them created by constant compression forces from the weight of the body being supported in poor postures. This discussion will focus on the most common type of lumbar disk pathology - disk degeneration leading to herniation and rupture with subsequent pressure on spinal nerves. The intervertebral disk is constantly exposed to compressive forces. This constant pressure over time will cause the fibers of the annulus fibrosis to break down. As these fibers break down, the nucleus pulposus inside the disk will press against the side of the disk. This will cause the disk to protrude and lose its circular shape. If the protrusion is severe and the annulus fibers break down all the way to the edge of the disk, the nucleus pulposus will escape from the disk and into the spinal canal.

The nucleus material is somewhat spongy so it is not immediately absorbed by the body. It may press on a nerve root or the dura mater causing radiating pain down the length of the nerve.

Figure 7-8b
Protrusion of an intervertebral disk which presses on a nerve.
(Illustration courtesy of Educational Graphics)

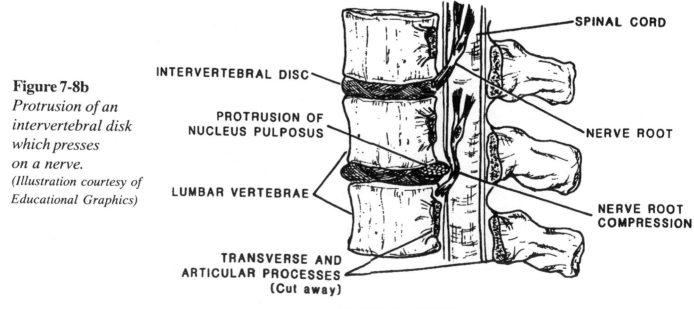

LATERAL VIEW

116

ASSESSMENT: The nature of back pain is that it's still very hard to pinpoint exactly where the problem is coming from. Often more specific diagnostic tests such as a myelogram, X-Ray, or MRI may be needed in order to be more certain of the nature of the pathology. In some instances information gained from physical examination may be helpful in determining the nature of the condition. With disk protrusions that are causing pain down the leg there are several characteristics that the practitioner may want to watch for. Pain from disk problems tends to be worse when sitting for long periods. Disk compression is greatest when in the sitting position. Movements in one direction may aggravate the pain and a slight change in the movement may relieve the pain. This will happen as the pressure is relieved on the nerve by slightly changing the position of each vertebral segment. With back pain that is the result of disk pathology, pain seems to decrease with activity. With back pain that is of a muscular origin, pain will usually increase with activity. Some clarification may be gained by performing the straight leg raise test.

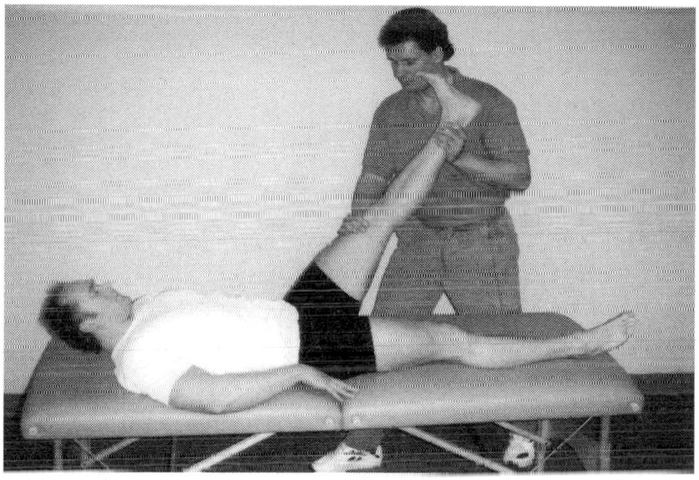

Figure 7-8c
The straight leg raise test

STRAIGHT LEG RAISE TEST- The client is supine on the treatment table. The therapist will bring the client's straight leg into flexion (if pain is radiating down the leg, use the leg which the pain is going down). Bring the leg up until the point of pain is reached that recreates the pain the client is feeling. This pain may be localized to the lumbar region or it may go down the leg. When the point of pain is reached, lower the leg about 2 inches. At that point, have the client dorsiflex the foot. Ask whether this motion has caused increased pain. The purpose in dorsiflexing the foot is to stretch the sciatic nerve and dura mater to see if it then presses against a disk protrusion. This will reproduce the client's pain. If this does not reproduce the pain, a little more stretch can be added to the dura mater by having the client slightly flex the neck as if picking their head up off the table. Again make note if this causes the pain symptoms to increase. If pain is increased with any of these moves, it is likely that there is involvement from a lumbar disk.

SUGGESTIONS FOR TREATMENT: There are a variety of ways to address lumbar disk protrusions. Vigorous arguments and debates abound in the health care field about the best way to treat them. Some of the options include surgery (which appears best used only in the most severe cases), manipulation or mobilization of the vertebral segments, traction, special exercises, or symptomatic treatments aimed at reducing pain. Massage therapy may be effective with this type of condition through an indirect approach. Massage will have little or no direct effect on the actual disk herniation or protrusion. However, if excessive compressive forces of the lumbar vertebra are causing the disk herniation, massage may be helpful. Many of the muscles attaching to the transverse and spinous processes of the lumbar spine become tight in reaction to the pain. This tightness increases the compression on the disk and may aggravate the condition. Releasing tightness on theses muscles is an indirect way to interrupt the cycle of pain and muscle tightness causing the compression.

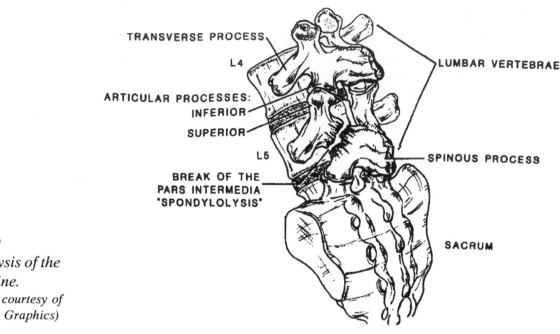

TRANSVERSE PROCESS

L4

LUMBAR VERTEBRAE

ARTICULAR PROCESSES:
INFERIOR
SUPERIOR

L5

SPINOUS PROCESS

BREAK OF THE
PARS INTERMEDIA
'SPONDYLOLYSIS'

SACRUM

POSTEROLATERAL VIEW

Figure 7-9
Spondylolysis of the
lumbar spine.
(Illustration courtesy of
Educational Graphics)

CHARACTERISTICS: Spondylolysis literally means the breakdown of the vertebral structure. This condition also develops as a result of compressive forces on the vertebra. It often originates with a break-down of a small section of the vertebra known as the pars interarticularis (noted as pars intermedia in Figure 7-9). As the vertebrae are compressed together there is a slackening of the posterior longitudinal ligament which runs along the sides of the vertebral bodies. The slackening of this ligament allows further disk protru-sion and may also trap protruding disk material between the bodies of the vertebrae and the slackened ligament. Eventually this disk material may ossify and become a bone spur. Nerve roots are then subject to being pressed as they drag across the bone spur formation. Also as a result of this breakdown of the vertebral structure is the narrowing of the intervertebral foramen, the space between the vertebra where the spinal nerves exit the spinal canal. When the vertebrae are pressed closer together and this channel narrows, it increases the possibility that there will be some type of nerve compression in the foramen. When the vertebrae are compressed together it is also likely to lead to irritation of the facet joints, the articulating surfaces of the adjacent vertebrae.

ASSESSMENT: Spondylolysis is usually associated with general degenerative changes in the spine which may be the result of age or chronic compression. Some factors in the history may point to its presence, but it will be most accurately identified through X-Ray.

SUGGESTIONS FOR TREATMENT: Reduction of the compressive forces on the vertebrae is of primary concern. In some instances rest and stretching will be indicated. Massage is likely to be helpful in reducing muscular components of the compression and biomechanical imbalance between individual verte-bral segments.

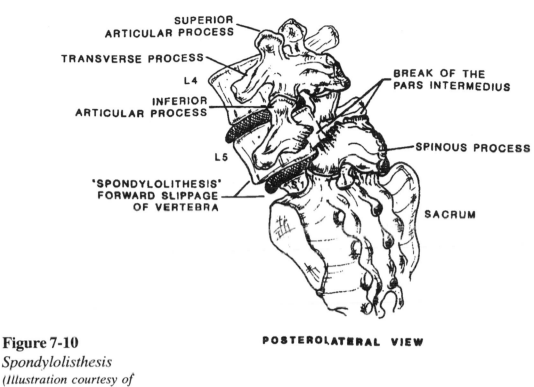

SUPERIOR
ARTICULAR PROCESS

TRANSVERSE PROCESS

L4

INFERIOR
ARTICULAR PROCESS

L5

'SPONDYLOLITHESIS'
FORWARD SLIPPAGE
OF VERTEBRA

BREAK OF THE
PARS INTERMEDIUS

SPINOUS PROCESS

SACRUM

POSTEROLATERAL VIEW

Figure 7-10
Spondylolisthesis
(Illustration courtesy of
Educational Graphics)

CHARACTERISTICS: The clinical characteristics of spondylolisthesis may be very similar to those of spondylolysis. In this condition the problem is caused by one vertebra slipping forward in relation to another. This most often happens at the L5-S1 junction. As the vertebra slips forward there is irritation to the facet joints and pain may be produced by increased tension on soft-tissue structures which are trying to hold the vertebra in place.

ASSESSMENT: As with spondylolysis, symptomatic complaints may indicate the presence of this condition. There may be an increased lumbar lordosis, which drives the lower lumbar vertebra in an anterior direction. This condition will be most accurately assessed by X-Ray examination.

SUGGESTIONS FOR TREATMENT: Treatment for spondylolisthesis will most often be through conservative measures such as rest, stretching exercises, and strengthening certain muscle groups that will help to reestablish proper mechanical alignment. Massage therapy may be helpful in achieving these objectives. However, deep massage treatment should be done with great caution, and any massage techniques that involve significant compression on the lumbar vertebra are not indicated.

(58) CONDITION: FACET JOINT IRRITATION

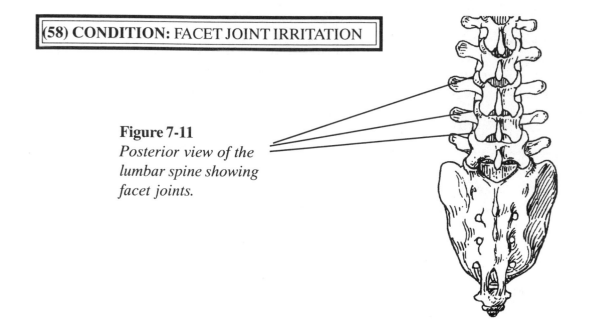

Figure 7-11
Posterior view of the lumbar spine showing facet joints.

CHARACTERISTICS: The facet joints (zygopophyseal joints) of the vertebra are the only location where adjacent vertebrae articulate with each other. Because of the mobility required of the spine and the unique shape of the vertebrae, this poses interesting problems for the mechanical structure of the facet joints. Back conditions which involve compression of adjacent vertebra will often irritate the facet joints. Just as improper mechanical irritation would cause pain, irritation, and degenerative changes at any other joint, it may happen at the facet joints as well. Pain will often be referred to other regions such as the coccyx, sacrum, gluteal region, or groin. Pain will usually be associated with motion.

ASSESSMENT: Facet joint irritation may often be difficult to determine. There are many other conditions which mimic its symptoms. Most clients with facet joint irritation will report pain that appears localized close to the midline of the spine. The pain is likely to be present with both active and passive motion. Pain will often be relieved with rest, but may become worse as the person gets up to move around. Muscles around the irritated facet may also be in spasm in an attempt to guard against the movement which is causing the pain.

SUGGESTIONS FOR TREATMENT: There are a number of treatment options that may help take pressure off the facet joints and decrease the irritation such as manipulation or mobilization of the joints. Instruction in postural mechanics will often be helpful. It is frequently the activities that a person performs every day that primarily lead to the development of this condition. Manual traction techniques will often be helpful to relieve the compression of the facet joints. Massage techniques directed at relieving the tight spinal extensor muscles will also be indicated. Stretching and the use of any modalities that can relieve muscle tightness will also help.

(59) CONDITION: MUSCLE STRAIN

CHARACTERISTICS: Acute or chronic overloading of musculotendinous structures in the lumbar and thoracic spine will lead to muscle strains. Because of the postural stress placed on these regions, muscle strains are relatively frequent. There is debate in some of the medical literature about the frequency of muscle strains involved in low back pain. However, clinical experience of manual therapists appears to indicate a relatively high proportion of problems originating from soft-tissues, many of them muscle strains. Muscle strains occur most often from excessive eccentric loading. This happens frequently to back muscles when a person bends down to pick something up. It may only be something as light as a pencil and then their back "goes out". This often occurs because the back extensor muscles have been overloaded to just under the point of fatigue. It is that one little next move that pushes them over the limit. Despite the frequency of muscle strains to the back, it is often difficult to pinpoint which exact muscles have the problem because so many of the postural muscles of the spine are quite small. This is one area in which skills of palpation become highly important.

ASSESSMENT: Knowledge of anatomy will be crucial in determining the presence of muscle strains. These conditions may have a number of symptoms depending on their severity. See the section in the beginning of the book on muscle strains for a more complete description of the differences between the various grades of strain. Determination of muscle pain or weakness may be based on the use of various manual resistive tests which isolate that muscle. Manual resistive tests for the movements of the lumbar and thoracic spine were included at the beginning of this chapter. Because of the difficulty in positioning, some manual resistive tests may be hard to perform. In many instances you will have to rely on information that the client gives you about what movements cause pain and discomfort and use that information to determine what muscles are being aggravated. It is often reported that you can be about 75-80% sure of what is the nature of the client's problem if you take an accurate history.

SUGGESTIONS FOR TREATMENT: Any discussion of the treatment of muscle strains must be considered relative to the degree of the strain. For instance, the method of treatment for a grade 1 strain will be different from that of a severe grade 3 strain. In most instances, muscle strains will be treated with rest from the offending activity, some type of anti-inflammatory treatment, stretching in the post-acute phase, and gradual strengthening as the injury repair progresses. Massage applications such as deep transverse friction are quite effective in helping to create a functional scar that is strong, yet pliable enough not to impair proper use of the tissue. Massage is also very helpful during the rehabilitative phase to decrease muscle spasm which may have occurred immediately after the injury and is preventing the proper biomechanical balance from returning. This will be especially important for the muscles of the spine which are predominantly postural muscles. Their role in maintaining posture during daily activity often makes it difficult to rest them appropriately. In addition, fibrosity following a muscle strain may often occur because that muscle is held in a shortened position for a prolonged period (such as with sitting at a desk all day). In this instance therapeutic intervention such as massage or stretching will be an invaluable method for returning proper function to the muscle.

---

(60) CONDITION: NEUROMUSCULAR PAIN

CHARACTERISTICS: Any muscle in the body is capable of holding an increased level of neurological activity and maintaining a spasm. The spasm of that muscle will then lead to increased pain and disturbed biomechanical function. This is especially true for the postural muscles of the spine. Muscle spasm can be perpetuated by various stimuli including chemicals like caffeine, certain medications, myofascial trigger points, or emotional stress. Muscular pain in the lumbar and thoracic spine that is the result of trigger point activity is often under reported or misdiagnosed as various joint pathologies. The pain may be relieved by rest, but simple activities of daily living will often cause the pain to resurface. Myofascial trigger points will often present with a confusing array of signs and symptoms for someone who is not on the lookout for them.

121

It is beneficial for the therapist to be aware of common reference zones of myofascial trigger points to determine if they are involved in each individual condition. These trigger points will often develop as a secondary manifestation to some other injury. For example, it is relatively common for clients who have lower extremity injuries to develop trigger points and muscle spasm in the muscles of the back. This happens as a result of postural adaptations to the change in gait.

ASSESSMENT: The muscles will frequently be painful in certain areas to palpation, may demonstrate a decreased range of motion, and may be somewhat painful on a resisted isometric contraction or stretching. They may contain painful myofascial trigger points which refer pain or other autonomic phenomena to remote areas. Chronic overuse, postural or biomechanical imbalances which are evident through the history may be indicating factors. See the sections above for references on manual resistive tests and range of motion testing for selected muscles of the lumbar and thoracic spine.

SUGGESTIONS FOR TREATMENT: These conditions respond very favorably to massage applications. Since muscular spasm is a primary component of these conditions, a technique like massage that is highly effective in addressing muscular spasm or trigger points is very effective in reducing the complaint. If the condition arises from poor postural or biomechanical function, movement reeducation is very helpful, and in most cases necessary, as an adjunctive treatment. The postural muscles of the spine are generally not strong or powerful muscles. Yet they have constant demands of heavy loading placed on them. Helpful suggestions of body mechanics will go a long way to making any treatment more effective. The use of heat or cold modalities where appropriate will also benefit these conditions.

Quick Reference for Conditions of the Lumbar & Thoracic Spine

REGION OF PAIN	ONSET	POSSIBLE CAUSE	REF.
LOW BACK, DOWN LOWER EXTREMITY	CHRONIC	LUMBAR DISK PATHOLOGY	55
ALONG SPINE, LOW BACK	CHRONIC	SPONDYLOLYSIS	56
ALONG SPINE, LOW BACK	CHRONIC	SPONDYLOLISTHESIS	57
ALONG SPINE, LOW BACK	CHRONIC	FACET JOINT IRRITATION	58
ANY MUSCLE	ACUTE OR CHRONIC	MUSCLE STRAIN	59
ANY MUSCLE	CHRONIC	NEUROMUSCULAR PAIN	60

CHAPTER 8

CERVICAL SPINE CONDITIONS

SPECIAL TERMS AND CONCEPTS

See the section on special terms and concepts for the lumbar and thoracic spine. The terms are used in the discussion of the cervical spine as well.

Overview of Common Single Plane Movements of the Cervical Spine

Active and passive ROM tests and manual resistive tests will require a knowledge of basic joint mechanics and functional anatomy for the regions surrounding the joint. The practitioner must know what constitutes normal, pain free motion in order to determine if there is a problem. The discussions of active ROM tests, passive ROM tests, and manual resistive tests will utilize the terms listed below. Familiarity with these terms and how they apply to the body will be essential in order to gain valid information from the assessment. All joint angle measurements which are included are measured from the neutral position, which is anatomical position. In order to properly understand and simplify joint mechanics, the movements at the joints described below have been broken down into single plane movements. That means movement in one of the three primary planes of motion - sagittal, frontal, or transverse. Although this greatly simplifies the analysis of movement it should be kept in mind that this classification rarely happens in actual human movement. Almost every movement we make will be a combination of movements in different planes. However, muscle or joint dysfunction can often be accurately pinpointed by comparing certain single plane movements. The primary muscles involved with each action are listed under the description of that action. Note that this may not include every muscle which is involved in that action, but only the primary ones. It should be noted that movements of the spine differ from movements of many other areas of the body in that movement is not occurring in one particular joint. The movements created in the spine are happening as a result of small degrees of movement between each of the individual vertebral segments. It is difficult to isolate motion at individual vertebral segments in the spine.

Flexion- this is a movement of the neck and head which brings the chin down toward the chest. Average range of motion in flexion is 80^0. The primary muscles involved with flexion are:

Rectus Capitis Anterior
Rectus Capitis Lateralis
Longus Capitis
Sternocleidomastoid
Longus Coli
Scalenes (Anterior, Medial, & Posterior)

Extension- a movement of the head which returns the head to anatomical position from a flexed position. When the head continues past anatomical position in the direction of extension it is considered hyperextension. Average range of motion in extension is 60^0 to 70^0. The primary muscles used in extension are:

Splenius Capitis
Semispinalis Capitis
Longissimus Capitis
Spinalis Capitis
Trapezius
Splenius Cervicis
Longissimus Cervicis
Semispinalis Cervicis

Lateral Flexion- a movement of the head which occurs in the frontal plane. The head tilts to the side bringing the ear down toward the same side shoulder. Average range of motion in lateral flexion is 35^0 to 45^0. The primary muscles used in lateral flexion are:

Levator Scapulae
Splenius Cervicis
Iliocostalis Cervicis
Longissimus Cervicis
Semispinalis Cervicis
Multifidus
Scalenes
Sternocleidomastoid

Rotation- a movement of the cervical spine which turns the head to one side. Since it is the central axis of the body that is turning, rotation is considered to be to the left and right instead of medial or lateral. In the discussion of muscles which are involved with rotation, refer back to the terms and concepts in the lumbar and thoracic spine for the definitions of ipsilateral and contralateral rotation. Average range of motion in rotation is about 80^0 to each side. The primary muscles involved with rotation are:

Levator Scapulae (ipsilateral)
Splenius Cervicis (ipsilateral)
Iliocostalis Cervicis (ipsilateral)
Longissimus Cervicis (ipsilateral)
Multifidus (contralateral)
Scalenes (contralateral)
Sternocleidomastoid (contralateral)

Active Range of Motion Tests

Active range of motion tests for the cervical spine will include the four single plane movements described above. The movements of lateral flexion and rotation should be performed to each side. It may be easiest to perform them in either a standing or sitting position.

Passive Range of Motion Tests

In some instances passive range of motion tests for the cervical spine are difficult to get accurate information about because many clients have a hard time "letting go" of their neck in order to let true passive motion occur. It is best to make sure you have a comfortable yet firm hold on their head when performing these motions. Be very aware to make all motions be smooth and slow. The cervical region can be very fragile and some people have had bad experiences with practitioners who gave them sudden and unexpected movements to the cervical region. This may create undue muscle guarding. The end-feel for all the single plane movements of the neck is tissue stretch, with the possible exception of extension. If a person is relatively flexible in the anterior cervical muscles there is no natural anatomical limitation to (hyper)extension of the neck. It may be stopped as the back of the head encounters the upper shoulders. This is one of the reasons that injuries from whiplash can be so severe.

Manual Resistive Tests

The next section includes illustrations and descriptions of manual resistive tests for the four single plane movements of the cervical spine. Remember that each of these movements can be performed in either of the two ways described earlier to perform manual resistive tests.

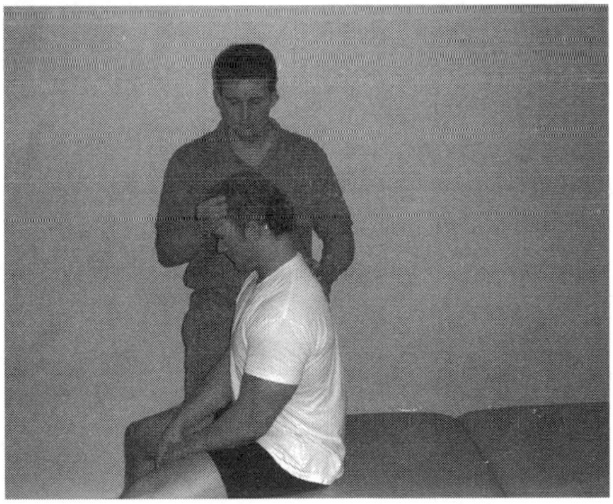

Figure 8-1
Resisted cervical flexion

The client is in a seated position on the treatment table. The therapist has one hand on the client's forehead and one hand on the upper back in order to help stabilize the upper torso and neck for movement. The head will be brought into a partial flexion. The client is instructed to try and bring the head down toward the chest while the therapist offers resistance.

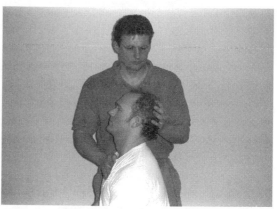

Figure 8-2
Resisted cervical extension

The client is in a seated position on the treatment table. The therapist has one hand on the back of the client's head and the other hand on the client's upper chest. The head will be brought back into a partial hyperextension. The client will be instructed to tilt the head back while the therapist offers resistance.

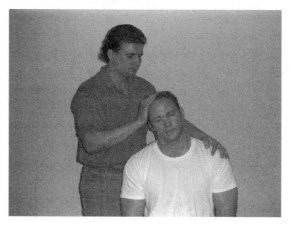

Figure 8-3
Resisted lateral flexion of the neck

The client is in a seated position and the therapist is standing at the client's side. The therapist will place one hand on the side of the client's head and the other hand on the opposite shoulder in order to stabilize the upper torso for movement. The head will be brought into a partial lateral flexion. The client will be instructed to hold the head in this position as the therapist attempts to move the head back into an upright position.

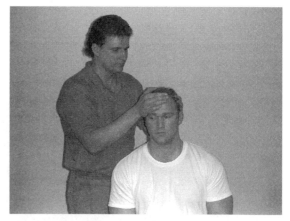

Figure 8-4
Resisted cervical rotation

The client is in a seated position. The therapist has one hand on the client's forehead and one hand on the client's occiput. The client will be instructed to hold the head in this position while the therapist attempts to rotate it in the opposite direction.

Structural and Postural Distortions

(61) CONDITION: FORWARD HEAD POSTURE

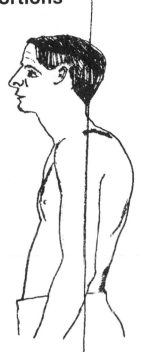

Figure 8-5
*Forward head posture which
puts stress on posterior
cervical muscles*

FOUND W/KYPHOSIS

CHARACTERISTICS: This postural condition is often present in conjunction with kyphosis, which was mentioned in the last chapter. The head is a heavy weight that is supported on a small base of support (the atlas). Poor postural habits or activities which require the head to be held in flexion for long periods, like reading, will cause the client to develop postural adaptations in which the head remains held forward of the center line of gravity. When the head comes forward of the center line of gravity, the posterior cervical muscles involved with extension must try to offset the forward displacement of the head. This makes these muscles constantly under stress. Since this position is likely to be held for a long period, these posterior cervical muscles will be subjected to prolonged tension. They will often develop chronic spasm and myofascial trigger points as a result.

ASSESSMENT: This condition is best assessed from a lateral view. It is beneficial to examine the client with a vertical reference such as a grid on the wall or a plumb line if possible. The ear should be close to a vertical line with the shoulder. If the head is significantly forward of this position, it is likely that the client is making postural adaptations to this forward head posture.

SUGGESTIONS FOR TREATMENT: In most instances this is a postural condition that has developed over a long period of time. It is not likely that you will be able to make a quick change. A slow, steady, progressive approach is far more likely to be successful. Massage applications should be directed at all the cervical musculature, but primarily at the posterior cervical muscles. Movement reeducation and postural awareness exercises such as those that are given in the Feldenkrais system or Alexander technique will be very helpful. It may be beneficial to tell the client to envision that the head is being held as if suspended from above and to imagine bringing the head up and back whenever he/she can be aware of it.

(62) CONDITION: RETRACTED HEAD POSTURE (MILITARY NECK)

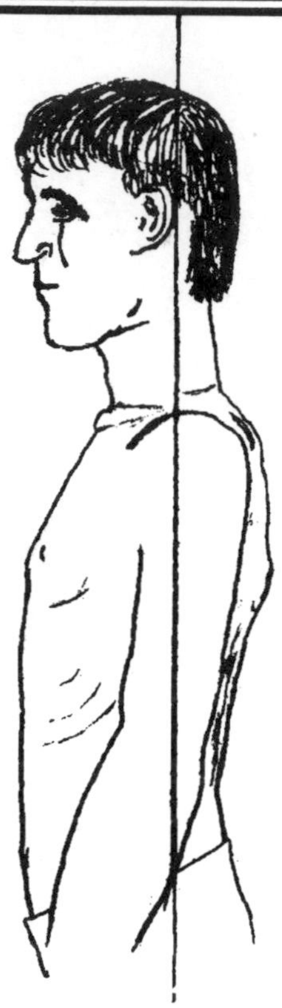

Figure 8-6
Retracted head posture of "military neck"

CHARACTERISTICS: There is a natural lordotic curve to the cervical region that is convex in an anterior direction just like the one in the lumbar region. This curve is necessary for proper weight distribution, shock absorption, and efficient movement of the head and neck. In a retracted head posture the lordotic cervical curve is lost and the vertebrae become stacked straight upon one another. This may lead to cervical vertebra or disk pathology as the compressive forces on the cervical vertebrae are compounded.

ASSESSMENT: This posture is best examined from a lateral direction. A wall grid or plumb line will be helpful. Look at the relationship of the neck to the shoulders in the normal relaxed standing position. There should be a natural slight lordotic curvature to the neck. If the posterior aspect of the neck appears straight and the person looks as if they are standing with a "stiff neck" they may have lost this lordotic curvature. This type of posture was often encouraged by military personnel. That is where the name comes from.

SUGGESTIONS FOR TREATMENT: This condition usually involves a lack of mobility in the cervical region. The vertical stacking of the vertebrae may lead to other cervical pathology. Stretching and massage to the posterior cervical muscles is encouraged. Massage approaches should address all the cervical musculature in order to achieve ideal balance. Some movement reeducation such as the type suggested for the forward head posture may also help.

WRONG — TREAT FRONT MUSCLES

Common Injury Conditions

---

(63) CONDITION: THORACIC OUTLET SYNDROME

---

scalene muscles

brachial plexus

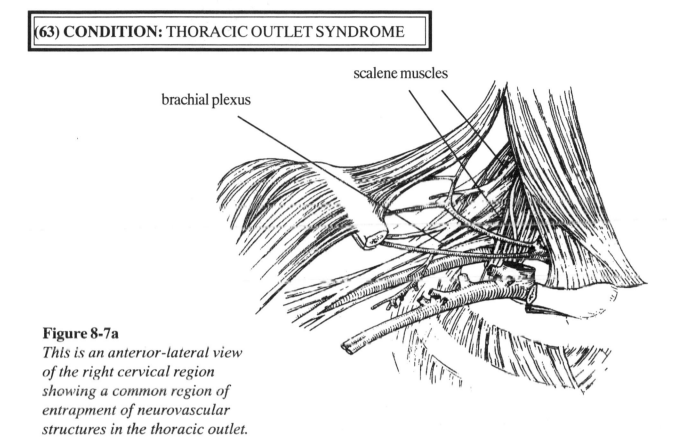

Figure 8-7a
*This is an anterior-lateral view
of the right cervical region
showing a common region of
entrapment of neurovascular
structures in the thoracic outlet.*

CHARACTERISTICS: Thoracic outlet syndrome is one of several common nerve impingement syndromes. The region between the anterior and medial scalene muscles where the nerves of the brachial plexus exit the neck is known as the thoracic outlet. In some medical literature this region is also called the thoracic inlet. If the anterior and medial scalene muscles are tight, they may press on nerve structures in the thoracic outlet. In addition to pressing on nerve structures, they may also press on vascular structures such as the subclavian artery. Symptoms will usually be pain, numbness, or paresthesia down the arm. Thoracic outlet syndrome is often sub-clinical (meaning not enough to cause any aggravating symptoms that the client is aware of) for long periods and some other type of neck or shoulder injury will cause it to become a primary problem.

ASSESSMENT: The client with thoracic outlet syndrome will usually have tight scalene muscles. There is often poor postural compensations that may involve the shoulders as well. The presence of thoracic outlet syndrome can be investigated in an indirect manner. The primary problem is impingement of the brachial plexus that is causing pain to go down the arm. In many instances when compression of the brachial plexus is present, so is compression of the subclavian artery. This can be examined through the use of the Adson maneuver.

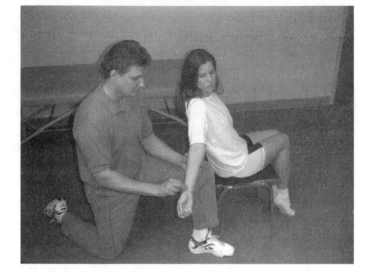

Figure 8-7b
Adson maneuver to examine for thoracic outlet syndrome.

ADSON MANEUVER- The client is in a seated position. The therapist will locate the radial pulse on the affected side. The radial pulse can be found on the anterior surface of the wrist just medial to the styloid process of the radius. Once the radial pulse is located, the therapist will bring the client's shoulder into extension and lateral rotation to the approximate position that is illustrated in Figure 8-7b. The client will turn the head as if looking over the affected shoulder. Once in this position, the client is instructed to take a deep breath. If the radial pulse diminishes or disappears it is likely that there is compression of the neurovascular structures in the thoracic outlet. Compression may also be created if the client looks over the opposite shoulder. The problem may be sub-clinical, in which case the diminishing of the pulse will indicate a predisposition to developing further problems with this condition.

SUGGESTIONS FOR TREATMENT: A multifaceted treatment approach is beneficial for this condition. Stretching of the scalene muscles and decreasing muscular imbalance in the cervical muscles will be of prime importance. Massage can be very effective in dealing with this condition. Caution should be used when addressing the scalene muscles with massage. Pressure in this area can directly compress the brachial plexus causing the aggravating symptoms to be intensified. As with many other approaches, knowledge of anatomy will be crucial to make your treatment specific and effective. Various muscle energy technique procedures or stretching may also be helpful for relieving tension in the cervical muscles.

(64) CONDITION: WHIPLASH

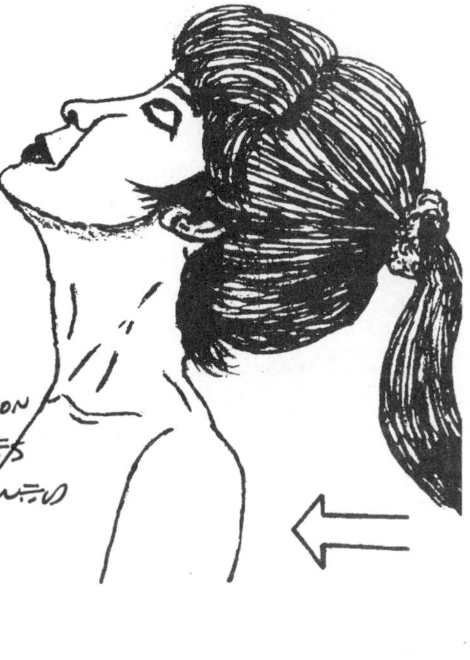

Figure 8-8
Whiplash- a sudden hyperextension of the cervical spine as a result of an impact from the rear indicated by the arrow. SUDDEN HYPER EXTENSION OF ANTERIOR /POSTERIOR MUSCLES OVER STRETCHING MUSCLE FOLLOWED BY FORCED COMPRESSION

132

CHARACTERISTICS: Whiplash is a common term that is used to describe a rapid back and forth movement that happens to the cervical region. This condition occurs most frequently in automobile accidents. Because the head is a heavy object balanced over a small base of support, the muscles of the cervical region are often subject to strong forces in trying to maintain the position of the head in violent accidents. Muscle spasm and pain will often develop following the injury. In some instances the muscle spasm and pain does not occur immediately, but may set in days later. The main part of the problem in whiplash occurs because of the rapid movement of the head following impact. The muscle spindles, which are the proprioceptors sensitive to the rate of changing length of a muscle, are highly activated with the rapid muscle lengthening that happens in whiplash. They may then cause reflex muscle spasms which will persist for long periods. Whiplash may also involve impingement of spinal nerves or cervical spinal cord injury as well.

ASSESSMENT: There is no specific clinical definition of whiplash. Therefore identifying it precisely is difficult. The most prominent symptoms will be a history of a violent movement of the neck followed either immediately or shortly afterward with significant muscle spasms. Active and passive range of motion will be limited and it is likely that manual resistive tests for numerous motions of the neck will be painful. Since many neck muscles have multiple actions, the whiplash is likely to affect most all of the neck muscles in some way.

SUGGESTIONS FOR TREATMENT: Treatment for whiplash will vary with the severity and the accompanying problems. Addressing the primary muscle spasm is a priority. This can be accomplished with cold applications and rest from any movements that increase discomfort. Because the likelihood for serious injury to neurological structures is high, it is a good idea for the client to have an evaluation by a physician in order to rule out more serious pathology. If the primary problem is with neck muscle spasm, massage applications can be very helpful. After the acute phase of the injury, use of heat modalities may be helpful to create a sense of pain relief and to enhance relaxation. *IF INDICATORS ARE SEVERE HAVE CLIENT GET X RAY (IN ACUTE PHASE)*

---

(65) CONDITION: TORTICOLLIS

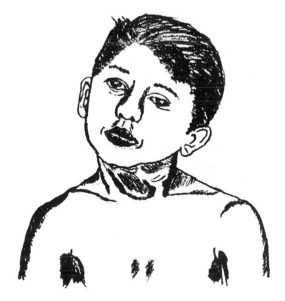

Figure 8-9
The extended and rotated position of the head characteristic of torticollis

CHARACTERISTICS: Torticollis is also frequently called wry neck. It is characterized by an acute muscle spasm of the posterior cervical muscles that may bring the head into slight extension and rotation to one side. Moving the head out of that position becomes painful and difficult. A person will often develop torticollis from sleeping in the wrong position and the muscles go into an acute spasm as a result of it.

ASSESSMENT: Torticollis will be evident if the client presents with a muscle spasm of the posterior cervical muscles that is of recent onset. The head will usually be inclined slightly upwards and to one side. There may be a precipitating trauma which happened before the muscle spasm occurred or it may have occurred in conjunction with other factors such as systemic illness, cold drafts, or sleeping in an awkward position. There will often be prominence of the sternocleidomastoid muscle on one side, as this is one of the primary muscles that is in spasm. *No- LEVATOR SCAPULA*

SUGGESTIONS FOR TREATMENT: Since torticollis involves muscle spasm as a primary component, massage applications are often quite helpful. The massage intervention must be of a low enough intensity not to induce further muscle spasm. Heat applications may be helpful when applied before the massage is performed. Some inhibitory stretching procedures such as the stretching techniques using the neurological principle of reciprocal inhibition may also be successful.

---

(66) CONDITION: CERVICAL DISK PATHOLOGY

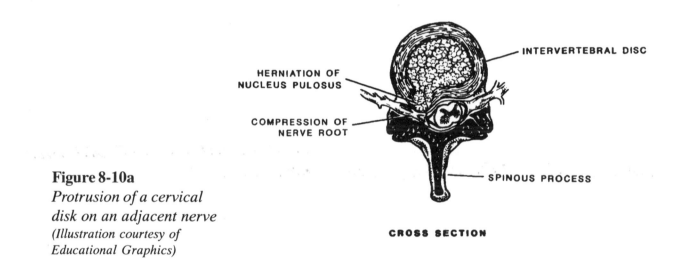

Figure 8-10a
Protrusion of a cervical disk on an adjacent nerve
(Illustration courtesy of Educational Graphics)

CHARACTERISTICS: This condition is very similar in development to the various lumbar disk pathologies described in chapter 7. See the discussion on lumbar disk pathologies in order to get a more thorough explanation of the breakdown of the intervertebral disk. When a cervical disk breaks down there are likely to be symptoms in the neck, head, arms, upper back, or shoulders. Cervical disk pathology can be especially difficult to isolate because of the many different movements and greater range of motion possible in the cervical region. This greater range of motion also makes the cervical region vulnerable to trauma forces. In addition, the size of the cervical vertebrae are much smaller than the lumbar vertebrae so their ability to withstand various forces is diminished.

ASSESSMENT: Any time there is pain in the neck, head, arms, or shoulders, the possibility of cervical disk involvement should be considered. This is a serious pathology that needs to be properly investigated. If a cervical disk pathology is present and the practitioner does not adequately screen for it, he/she may engage the client in various techniques or procedures such as stretching or range of motion activities that could make the condition worse. A client with cervical disk pathology will often report sharp, shooting pain down the arms or in the neck and shoulder region. This pain can usually

134

be reproduced by either active or passive motion. In most instances a manual resistive test from a neutral position would not engage the same pain. However, it might because of the muscular forces which are applied to the fragile structures of the neck. It is also important for the therapist to remember when asking the client if any testing procedure causes pain to make sure that it is the same pain they are accustomed to feeling. In some instances a special testing procedure may cause pain, but it is a different pain than the one that they feel during normal daily activities. In this instance you should consider that you have found something that may be a significant problem. However, it may not be the problem that you are looking for. Involvement of cervical disk pathology may sometimes become apparent with the use of compression or distraction tests because of their effect on opening or closing the narrow space where the nerves exit the vertebrae.

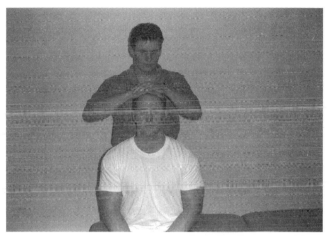

Figure 8-10b
Cervical compression examining for cervical disk pathology.

CERVICAL COMPRESSION- The client is in a seated position on the treatment table. The therapist will place both hands on top of the client's head. A slow gentle pressure will be applied pressing straight down on the top of the client's head. If the client reports any increase in pain or discomfort, it is likely that there is involvement with cervical disk pathology.

Figure 8-10c
Cervical traction examining for cervical disk pathology

CERVICAL TRACTION- The therapist is standing at the client's side. The client is in a seated position. The therapist will place one hand on the client's forehead and one hand behind the client's occiput. A slow a gentle traction (pulling) force will be applied straight upwards. If there is a relief of pain with this pulling motion, it is likely that there is some involvement with cervical disk pathology and the client should probably be referred for a more thorough evaluation.

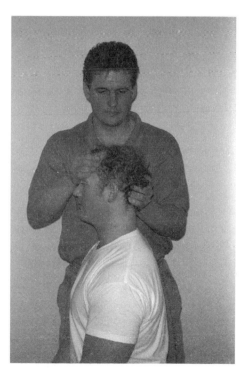

SUGGESTIONS FOR TREATMENT: Treatment for cervical disk pathology varies widely with the severity of the condition. Several conservative options that arc used include stretching and range of motion activities in order to restore proper muscular balance, therapeutic exercises, or home traction units (usually a water-filled bag on a pulley system that is hung over a door). Massage may be helpful for some cervical disk pathologies if the condition is not too severe. Muscular tension and imbalance may be a primary factor for the amount of compression on the cervical region. This can be adequately addressed through the use of massage. Various thermal modalities (heat or cold) may also be helpful where appropriate.

(67) CONDITION: MUSCLE STRAIN

CHARACTERISTICS: Acute or chronic overloading of musculotendinous structures in the cervical spine will lead to muscle strains. Because of the postural stress placed on these regions, muscle strains are relatively frequent. The fact that the head is supported over a narrow base of support and primarily held in place by muscles acting as "guy wires" will often lead to overloading of these muscles. Despite the frequency of muscle strains to the neck, it is often difficult to pinpoint which exact muscles are the primary cause of the problem because so many of the neck muscles have multiple movements. In addition many of these muscles, such as the sub-occipital muscle group are quite small.

ASSESSMENT: Knowledge of anatomy will be crucial in determining the presence of muscle strains. These conditions may have a number of symptoms depending on their severity. See the section in the beginning of the book on muscle strains for a more complete description of the differences between the various grades of strain. Determination of muscle pain or weakness may be based on the use of various manual resistive tests which isolate that muscle. Manual resistive tests for the movements of the cervical spine were included at the beginning of this chapter. It often takes very little effort in manual resistive tests of the cervical region to elicit symptoms if there is a muscle strain present. One of the most confusing factors with muscular problems in the cervical region is that muscles are often painful when both contracting and stretching over very short distances. It then becomes harder to tell which muscle is really causing the problem, and if it is painful because of contraction or elongation. The frequency of referred pain from neck muscles is another confounding factor that makes the identification of muscular problems of the neck difficult. For these reasons skilled palpation will become a crucial part of your assessment of cervical problems.

SUGGESTIONS FOR TREATMENT: Any discussion of the treatment of muscle strains must be considered relative to the degree of the strain. For instance, the method of treatment for a grade 1 strain will be different from that of a severe grade 3 strain. In most instances muscle strains will be treated with rest from the offending activity, some type of anti-inflammatory treatment, stretching in the post-acute phase, and gradual strengthening as the injury repair progresses. Massage applications such as deep transverse friction are quite effective in helping to create a functional scar that is strong, yet pliable enough not to impair that proper use of the tissue. However, because of positioning factors and the delicate structures in the cervical region, it is difficult to perform deep transverse friction in the cervical region. The therapist is then encouraged to modify the approach in order to accommodate these adjustments.

Massage is also very helpful during the rehabilitative phase to decrease muscle spasm which may have occurred immediately after the injury and is preventing the proper biomechanical balance from returning. This will be especially important for the muscles of the spine which are predominantly postural muscles. Their role in maintaining posture during daily activity often makes it difficult to rest them appropriately. In addition, fibrosity following a muscle strain may often occur because that muscle is held in a shortened position for a prolonged period (such as with sitting at a desk all day). In this instance therapeutic intervention such as massage or stretching will be an invaluable method for returning proper function to the muscle.

(68) CONDITION: NEUROMUSCULAR PAIN

CHARACTERISTICS: Any muscle in the body is capable of holding an increased level of neurological activity and maintaining a spasm. The spasm of that muscle will then lead to increased pain and disturbed biomechanical function. This is especially true for the postural muscles of the spine. Muscle spasm can be perpetuated by various stimuli including chemicals like caffeine, certain medications, myofascial trigger points, or emotional stress. Muscular pain in the cervical spine that is the result of trigger point activity is very common. The pain may be relieved by rest, but simple activities of daily living will often cause the pain to resurface. Myofascial trigger points will often present with a confusing array of signs and symptoms for someone who is not on the lookout for them. It is beneficial for the therapist to be aware of common reference zones of myofascial trigger points to determine if they are involved in each individual condition. These trigger points will often develop as a secondary manifestation to some other injury.

Headaches that are the result of muscular tension are frequent. The small sub-occipital muscles that are between the axis and the occiput are often the culprits. They are difficult to access which often makes chronic headaches a continuous problem for many people. Becoming familiar with the common reference zones of trigger points in the cervical region will be helpful in designing the most effective treatment approach for problems in this region.

ASSESSMENT: The muscles will frequently be painful in certain areas to palpation, may demonstrate a decreased range of motion, and may be somewhat painful on a resisted isometric contraction or stretching. They may contain painful myofascial trigger points which refer pain or other autonomic phenomena to remote areas. Chronic overuse, postural or biomechanical imbalances which are evident through the history may be indicating factors. See the sections above for references on manual resistive tests and range of motion testing for selected muscles of the cervical spine.

SUGGESTIONS FOR TREATMENT: These conditions respond very favorably to massage applications. Since muscular spasm is a primary component of these conditions, a technique like massage that is highly effective in addressing muscular spasm or trigger points is very effective in reducing the complaint. If the condition arises from poor postural or biomechanical function, movement reeducation is very helpful, and in most cases necessary, as an adjunctive treatment. The postural muscles of the spine are generally not strong or powerful muscles. Yet they have constant demands of heavy loading placed on them. Helpful suggestions of body mechanics will go a long way to making any treatment more effective. The use of heat or cold modalities where appropriate will also benefit these conditions.

Quick Reference for Conditions of the Cervical Spine

REGION OF PAIN	ONSET	POSSIBLE CAUSE	REF.
NECK, SHOULDER, OR ARM	CHRONIC	THORACIC OUTLET SYNDROME	63
NECK OR SHOULDERS	ACUTE	WHIPLASH	64
NECK OR SHOULDERS	ACUTE OR CHRONIC	TORTICOLLIS	65
NECK, HEAD, SHOULDER, ARM, OR HAND	ACUTE OR CHRONIC	CERVICAL DISK PATHOLOGY	66
ANY MUSCLE	ACUTE OR CHRONIC	MUSCLE STRAIN	67
ANY MUSCLE	CHRONIC	NEUROMUSCULAR PAIN	68

CHAPTER 9

SHOULDER CONDITIONS

Overview of Common Single Plane Movements of the Shoulder

Active and passive ROM tests and manual resistive tests will require a knowledge of basic joint mechanics and functional anatomy for the regions surrounding the joint. The practitioner must know what constitutes normal, pain free motion in order to determine if there is a problem. The discussions of active ROM tests, passive ROM tests, and manual resistive tests will utilize the terms listed below. Familiarity with these terms and how they apply to the body will be essential in order to gain valid information from the assessment. All joint angle measurements which are included are measured from the neutral position, which is anatomical position. In order to properly understand and simplify joint mechanics, the movements at the joints described in each regional section in the book have been broken down into single plane movements. That means movement in one of the three primary planes of motion - sagittal, frontal, or transverse. Although this greatly simplifies the analysis of movement it should be kept in mind that this classification rarely happens in actual human movement. Almost every movement we make will be a combination of movements in different planes. However, muscle or joint dysfunction can often be accurately pinpointed by comparing certain single plane movements. The primary muscles involved with each action are listed under the description of that action. Note that this may not include every muscle which is involved in that action, but only the primary ones.

Flexion- a movement of the shoulder in which it is brought straight up in front of the body moving in the sagittal plane. Average range of motion in flexion will usually go up all the way to 180^0. In some instances the individual may be able to go past 180^0. When the movement goes past full flexion at 180^0 it is called hyperflexion. The shoulder is the only joint in the body that can go into hyperflexion as part of its normal movement. The primary muscles involved in flexion are:

> **Anterior Deltoid**
> **Pectoralis Major**
> **Coracobrachialis**
> **Biceps Brachii**

Extension- a movement of the shoulder in the sagittal plane which returns it to anatomical position from any position of flexion. When the shoulder continues in the direction of extension past anatomical position, it is in hyperextension. Note that the amount of extension that is measured in the average range of motion is all in hyperextension. Average range of motion in extension is 45^0 to 50^0. The primary muscles involved in extension are:

> **Posterior Deltoid**
> **Teres Major**
> **Teres Minor**
> **Latissimus Dorsi**
> **Pectoralis Major**
> **Triceps (long head)**

Abduction- a movement of the shoulder which moves the arm in a frontal plane away from the midline of the body. Ironically, during the second half of the abduction movement as the arm is coming vertical it is once again moving toward the midline of the body. However this is still considered abduction. Average range of motion in abduction is 180^0. The primary muscles used in abduction are:

Deltoid
Supraspinatus
Infraspinatus (upper fibers)

Adduction- a movement of the shoulder in the frontal plane which brings the arm back to anatomical position from any amount of abduction. This movement brings the arm back toward the midline of the body. Average range of motion in adduction is 30^0 to 45^0. NOTE: This additional motion that is measured as 30^0 to 45^0 of abduction is done when combined with a slight degree of flexion. This brings the arm across the front of the torso. The torso prevents the arm from moving any further into adduction than anatomical position. The primary muscles used in adduction are:

Pectoralis Major   *INFRA SPANATUS*
Latissimus Dorsi
Teres Major
Subscapularis

Medial/Internal Rotation- a movement of the shoulder which rotates the arm around a vertical axis in the transverse plane toward the midline of the body. This is easiest to visualize if the elbow is brought into 90^0 of flexion so that the fingertips point straight ahead. The shoulder is then rotated so the forearm is now resting across the mid-torso. Average range of motion in medial/internal rotation is about 100^0. Note that the torso will prevent motion from occurring more than 90^0 if the elbow is in the reference position described. However if you reach behind your back (the shoulder is now in partial hyperextension), the remaining amount of internal rotation is possible. The primary muscles responsible for medial/internal rotation are:

Pectoralis Major
Anterior Deltoid
Latissimus Dorsi
Teres Major
Subscapularis

Lateral/External Rotation- a movement of the shoulder which rotates the arm around a vertical axis in the transverse plane away from the midline of the body. This is easiest to visualize if the elbow is brought into 90^0 of flexion so that the fingertips point straight ahead. The shoulder is then rotated so the forearm is now turning away from the body. Average range of motion in lateral/external rotation is about 80^0. The primary muscles involved in lateral/external rotation are:

Infraspinatus
Posterior Deltoid
Teres Minor

There are two additional movements which are mentioned at the shoulder because of its unique structure. The shoulder is really composed of several joints. Two of the joints are intimately connected with producing movement at the shoulder - the glenohumeral joint and the scapulothoracic articulation (it is called an articulation because it is not a true joint). Combined motion at the glenohumeral joint and the scapulothoracic articulation are capable of producing these two additional movements:

Horizontal Abduction- a movement in which the arm moves parallel to the ground in the transverse plane beginning in a position of 90^0 of abduction (out to the side). From this position the arm is brought further back as if the person is reaching behind him/herself. Average range of motion in horizontal abduction is 30^0. The primary muscles used in horizontal abduction are

> **Posterior Deltoid**
> **Teres Major**
> **Teres Minor**
> **Infraspinatus**

Horizontal Adduction- a movement in which the arm moves parallel to the ground in a transverse plane beginning in a position of 90^0 of abduction (out to the side). From this position the arm is brought across the front of the torso. Average range of motion in horizontal adduction is $140''$. The primary muscles involved in horizontal adduction are:

> **Pectoralis Major**
> **Anterior Deltoid**

Active Range of Motion Tests

Active range of motion tests for the shoulder will focus on the six primary single plane movements of the glenohumeral joint described above. The movements required by the shoulder in horizontal adduction and horizontal abduction will be covered through other motions of the six primary single plane movements. It may be easiest to perform them in a standing position.

Passive Range of Motion Tests

Because of the mobility of the shoulder joint and the complex network of soft-tissue structures, the nature of movement during passive motion is very important in determining the origin of a problem. The end-feel(s) for flexion, extension, medial, & lateral rotation will all be tissue stretch. The end-feel in adduction will be tissue approximation as the arm encounters the torso. The end-feel for abduction will be most like tissue stretch, but in certain individuals who have great flexibility, the motion may be halted by the head of the humerus encountering the acromion process, although this bone-to-bone encounter will not be as abrupt as the one at the end of elbow extension.

Manual Resistive Tests

The next section includes illustrations and descriptions of manual resistive tests for the six primary single plane movements of the shoulder joint. Remember that each of these movements can be performed in either of the two ways described earlier to perform manual resistive tests.

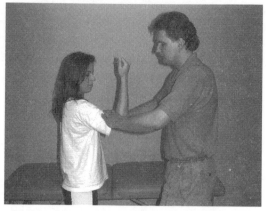

Figure 9-1
*Resisted flexion
of the shoulder*

The client is in a seated or standing position. With the arm forward flexed to approximately 90^0. The therapist will place both hands around the clients arm and the client will be instructed to attempt to hold the arm in this position as the therapist attempts to push it down into extension.

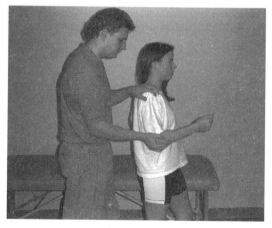

Figure 9-2
*Resisted extension
of the shoulder*

The client is in a standing position with the arm in a position close to neutral (anatomical position). The elbow is flexed to approximately 90^0. The therapist places one hand on the back of the client's elbow and the other hand on the shoulder to stabilize the torso and shoulder. The client will be instructed to attempt to further extend the arm while the therapist offers resistance.

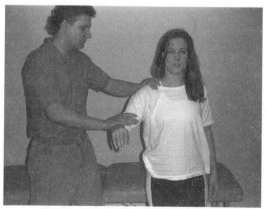

Figure 9-3
*Resisted abduction
of the shoulder*

The client is in a standing position with the arm abducted to about 45^0. The therapist places one hand on the lateral region of the elbow and the other hand on the shoulder to stabilize the shoulder and torso. The client will be instructed to hold the arm in this position as the therapist attempts to press the arm into adduction.

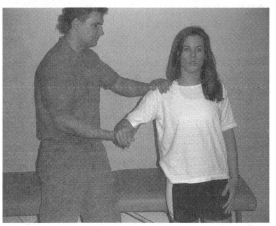

Figure 9-4
Resisted adduction
of the shoulder

The client is in the same position as that described for abduction. The arm is also in the same position. The therapist has one hand on the medial side of the client's elbow and one hand on the client's shoulder to stabilize the shoulder and torso. The client will be instructed to pull the arm in toward the body (or hold it in that position) while the therapist attempts to pull the arm out in abduction.

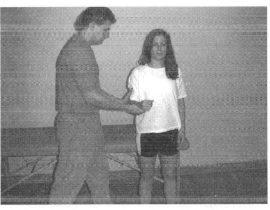

Figure 9-5
Resisted medial rotation
of the shoulder

The client is in a standing position with the elbow flexed to 90⁰. The flexion of the elbow helps give a lever for the rotation movement at the shoulder which is desired. The client will be instructed to keep the arm close to the body during the test. The therapist will have on hand on the inside of the client's wrist and one hand on the client's lateral elbow region to hold it against the body. The shoulder will be in a neutral forward position and the client will be instructed to hold the shoulder in this position as the therapist attempts to pull the wrist toward himself (in the direction of lateral rotation).

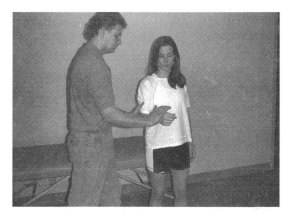

Figure 9-6
Resisted lateral rotation
of the shoulder

The client is in the same starting position as for medial rotation. The therapist will have one hand on the lateral elbow region and one hand on the outside of the client's wrist. The client will be instructed to hold the shoulder in this position as the therapist attempts to push the client's wrist toward her torso in the direction of medial rotation.

Structural and Postural Deviations

(69) CONDITION: ELEVATED SHOULDER

*LAT DORSI
LOWER TRAP
QL*

*✓ UPPER TRAP
LEVATOR SCAPULA*

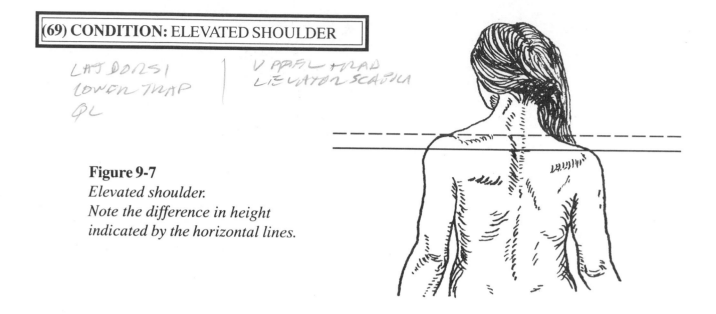

Figure 9-7
Elevated shoulder.
Note the difference in height
indicated by the horizontal lines.

CHARACTERISTICS: The shoulders are an area that generally hold a great deal of postural and emotional tension in the form of sustained muscular contractions. One of the most common areas for this to be evident is in the upper shoulder region with tension held in the upper trapezius and levator scapula muscles. This has the shoulders in a raised or "elevated" position compared to their normal location. This condition is seen frequently in people who spend long hours at a desk with their arms raised to rest on the desk. Working at various workstations for long hours will tend to make this posture happen as well. An example is working on a computer keyboard that is placed on a normal desk. The normal desk height is not designed to accommodate a computer keyboard and therefore the person must raise his/her shoulders to get the hands up to the level of the keyboard. This increased tension in the shoulder muscles will often lead to muscle tension headaches.

ASSESSMENT: One shoulder may be held higher than the other or both shoulders may elevated. This condition is best assessed by viewing the client from the front or back. If one shoulder is higher than the other it should be relatively easy to see the height difference. If both shoulders are high, however it becomes harder to tell if the shoulders are elevated or if that is the natural alignment for that individual. It will also be helpful to see if there is tightness of the shoulder elevator muscles such as the upper trapezius and the levator scapula.

SUGGESTIONS FOR TREATMENT: Since this is a condition that primarily involves muscular tension, massage applications are very helpful in addressing this problem. However, there is a postural component that is often directly related to the way in which each individual manifests stress in his/her body. That will also need to be addressed. Heat applications will generally be helpful to decrease muscle tension and make the massage treatments more effective. Stretching of the posterior cervical muscles and the lateral flexors will also be helpful. It is also beneficial to give the client some suggestions about postural modifications that can be done with daily activities that may be aggravating this condition.

Figure 9-8
Retracted shoulders.
Scapula are pulled together
in the back.

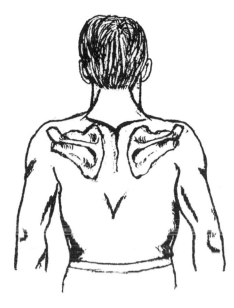

CHARACTERISTICS: This is a posture that is often exaggerated among military recruits, hence its name. When the two scapula are pulled back (sometimes called retraction or adduction), the rhomboid and middle trapezius muscles will be in a shortened position and usually tight. This limits proper mobility of the shoulder girdle. Since this condition involves an angulation and positioning of the scapula, it may have a detrimental effect on the mechanics of the glenohumeral joint causing other shoulder pathologies. This is because the angulation of the glenoid fossa is changed slightly when the scapula moves in any position. Even a very slight change in location or facing of the glenoid fossa can have serious ramifications for proper shoulder mechanics.

ASSESSMENT: This condition is best assessed by looking at the client from the front and the rear. From the front the client will have an appearance that the shoulders are being forcibly held back. There may be a visual sense that the chest is overinflated or being pushed out. From behind it will appear that the arms are being pulled back and the scapula are much closer to the spine than normal. There will likely be tightness in many different muscles of the shoulder girdle. The client may also present with symptoms of pain or paresthesia down the arm because the pectoralis minor muscle may be entrapping the brachial plexus against the upper rib cage. (See reference #76 on pectoralis minor syndrome in this chapter).

SUGGESTIONS FOR TREATMENT: This condition often involves significant muscular spasm which can be addressed by massage. Massage applications should focus on the upper thoracic muscles such as the rhomboids and middle trapezius, but all muscles of the shoulder girdle should be addressed. Stretching exercises in which the shoulder and arm are brought into horizontal adduction are also likely to help. This can be done by having the client bend over forward at the waist and hold a heavy object in the arm which is hanging toward the floor.

(71) CONDITION: FORWARD "SLUMPED" SHOULDERS

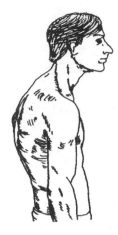

PEC MAJOR
PEC MINON
SCM
SCALENES

Figure 9-9
Slumped shoulder posture

CHARACTERISTICS: The postural condition of slumped shoulders is increasingly common with those individuals who work at a desk or have some work station which requires holding the arms out in front of them for long periods. This also seems to be an acquired postural habit that may have emotional as well as postural components. As with the retracted shoulder condition, various pathologies of the gleno-humeral joint will often accompany this condition as the facing direction of the glenoid fossa is altered. In this condition the fossa aims in a more anterior direction. This disturbs the proper biomechanical balance around the joint.

ASSESSMENT: This condition is best assessed from the front. The client will have shoulders that seem to droop. The natural position of the hands in the upright standing posture is at the sides. In the slumped shoulder posture the hands will hang to the anterior portion of the thigh. Because this condition also frequently involves a medial rotation of the shoulder along with the scapular angulation, the palms of the hands may face backwards as opposed to facing the thigh.

SUGGESTIONS FOR TREATMENT: This condition will usually benefit from a comprehensive approach that looks at postural, emotional and physical demands on the body. Massage treatment should be focused on helping to restore proper biomechanical balance to the area by decreasing tightness in the anterior shoulder girdle muscles. Stretching to these muscles will also be quite helpful. There are postural demands placed on the upper back muscles to hold the shoulder girdle in position while a person does work with the arms out in front. Therefore it is helpful to work on strengthening of the upper back and shoulder muscles that act on the posterior shoulder girdle such as the rhomboids, trapezius, latissimus dorsi, teres major & minor, and infraspinatus.

Common Injury Conditions

(72) CONDITION: SHOULDER SEPARATION

Figure 9-10a
Anterior view of the right shoulder. The line indicates the acromioclavicular ligament which is injured in a shoulder separation.

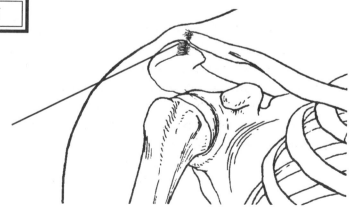

146

CHARACTERISTICS: A shoulder separation is characterized by a sprain to the acromioclavicular ligament. This sprain creates mobility of the acromioclavicular (A-C) joint. This condition frequently occurs from a fall directly on the shoulder. The force of the body weight landing on the acromion process or clavicle is greater than the strength of the ligament and it is torn. The clavicle acts primarily as a "strut" to the shoulder girdle so it is not in a particularly strong mechanical position. This is the common mechanism by which shoulder separations occur.

ASSESSMENT: The client will usually report some history of direct trauma to the shoulder joint. There is also likely to be specific joint tenderness at the A-C joint with possible swelling. If the injury is severe, visible dislocation of the distal end of the clavicle may be apparent. There is likely to be pain on a number of different movements. Most likely to cause pain is any movement, active or passive, which involves horizontal adduction. This is sometimes called the cross over test and is used to determine if there is an injury to the A-C joint.

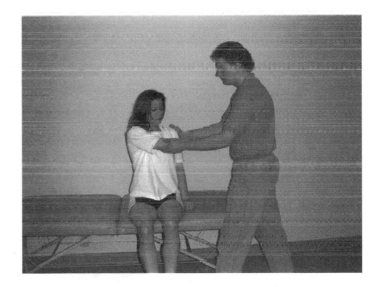

Figure 9-10b
Cross-over test examining for injury to the A-C joint

CROSS OVER TEST- The client is in a sitting or standing position. They will be asked to horizontally adduct the arm and bring it across the upper chest. The therapist may give a slight degree of additional pressure at the end range of motion as shown in Figure 9-10b. If there is significant injury to the A-C joint, it is likely that the client will have pain and discomfort with this movement.

SUGGESTIONS FOR TREATMENT: The injury will often be self-limiting, meaning a person will not do any activities that aggravate the condition. This will give it time to heal. It is best to avoid any movements of the shoulder in which the structures of the shoulder will be heavily loaded (such as lifting heavy weight or throwing). In the latter stages of the injury some strength training may be used in order to help strengthen the postural muscles around the shoulder which will be utilized to return stability to the area. If the injury is not severe, massage applications to the region of the A-C joint may also be helpful. Deep transverse friction may help produce a healthy and functional repair of the injured tissue. Massage is useful in helping to return optimum muscle function to the surrounding muscles. Very often, as a result of a local trauma, the muscles will go into spasm and disturb the mechanical balance around the joint.

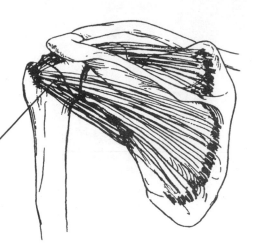

Figure 9-11a
Posterior view of the left shoulder. The line points to the conjoined tendons of the posterior rotator cuff, a common site of rotator cuff tearing.

CHARACTERISTICS: There can be a wide range of pathological conditions that fall under the category of rotator cuff tears. Because the rotator cuff muscle group is made up of four muscles: supraspinatus, infraspinatus, teres minor, and subscapularis, a strain to any of these muscles could be considered a rotator cuff tear. However, the most frequent problems with rotator cuff tears happen to the supraspinatus and infraspinatus. The supraspinatus muscle is often injured because of heavy mechanical demands placed on it during the motion of abduction. In addition it may be susceptible to chronic tearing of fibers from impingement underneath the acromion process. These chronic tears will frequently develop into long-term problems that can cause great pain and problems at the shoulder joint.

Rotator cuff tears also occur from constant eccentric loading. One example of how this frequently happens is the deceleration of the shoulder and arm in the follow through phase after throwing something. The big powerful muscles of the anterior shoulder girdle such as the pectoralis major and the anterior deltoid are responsible for generating acceleration of the throwing arm. It is the responsibility of the teres minor and infraspinatus along with a few others to slow down that motion during the follow through. This is a tremendous amount of force that these much smaller muscles are trying to decelerate. That is why the rotator cuff group are often torn.

ASSESSMENT: The best means of determining the presence of a rotator cuff tear from physical examination will be a careful mix of blending together information from the active, passive, and manual resistive tests of the different motions of the shoulder in conjunction with a thorough history. Rotator cuff tears may also present with tenderness at the distal portion of the supraspinatus tendon, the teres minor, or infraspinatus musculotendinous junctions. Remember that the rotator cuff muscles are a group, so a rotator cuff tear could be in any one of those muscles. If there is a severe rotator cuff tear which primarily affects the supraspinatus muscle it may show up with the drop arm test.

SHOWN THEW 40DO 1ST

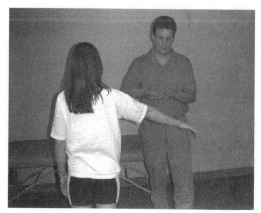

Figure 9-11b
The drop-arm test investigating for serious tears in the rotator cuff (primarily in supraspinatus)

DROP ARM TEST- The client is asked to abduct the arm to 90^0 and then slowly lower it back down. If a severe rotator cuff tear is present it is likely that she will not be able to smoothly lower the arm back down. It may, in fact, drop suddenly to her side. Another variation on this test is to have the client bring the arm up to 90^0 and then hold it there for a moment. The therapist will then lightly tap downward on the arm just over the wrist. If a severe rotator cuff tear is present, it is likely that the client will not be able to hold the arm in that position and the arm will drop to the side.

SUGGESTIONS FOR TREATMENT: There are a number of different ways to treat rotator cuff tears depending on their severity. A severe tear will often need to be treated with surgery. However, other conservative measures are often effective in gaining improvement. Strengthening other muscles of the shoulder girdle so that they can help in the mechanical demands is very useful. However, strengthening exercises which are engaged in too early may aggravate the problem more. It is most effective to address the soft-tissue injury with stretching, massage or some other treatment that will allow the damaged tissue to heal properly first. Deep transverse friction massage and some other methods that involve massage with active or passive motions will get good results. Stretching, mobilization and range of motion exercises can then be encouraged. Once a degree of tissue repair and flexibility have returned, strengthening is much more likely to be effective.

---

(74) CONDITION: SHOULDER IMPINGEMENT SYNDROME

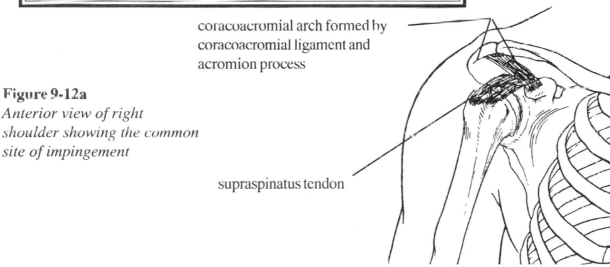

coracoacromial arch formed by coracoacromial ligament and acromion process

Figure 9-12a
Anterior view of right shoulder showing the common site of impingement

supraspinatus tendon

CHARACTERISTICS: There are a number of different tissue structures which may be at fault in shoulder impingement syndrome. There is a region in the shoulder joint called the coracoacromial arch. It is formed by the acromion process and the coracoacromial ligament. The supraspinatus tendon and the sub-acromial bursa are underneath this arch. Repeated abduction and forward flexion movements of the shoulder will impinge the supraspinatus tendon or sub-acromial bursa underneath the coracoacromial arch. This happens most often in clients who have to hold their arms in this position for long periods (like a house painter), or someone who engages in many repetitive motions of flexion and abduction (like a swimmer).

ASSESSMENT: Clients with shoulder impingement syndrome will most often report generalized pain just below the acromion process. Sometimes the pain may feel like it is deep in the shoulder joint. This pain will usually be aggravated with both passive and active range of motion activities at the end range of flexion or abduction. A history of repetitive overuse or chronic long periods of shoulder flexion or abduction will also be indicators. Additional information about the likelihood of shoulder impingement can also be gained from two special orthopedic tests- the empty can test and the Hawkins-Kennedy impingement sign.

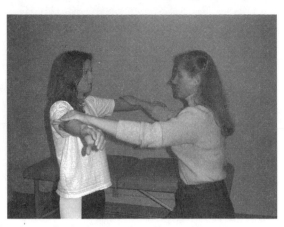

Figure 9-12b
The empty can test examining for shoulder impingement syndrome

EMPTY CAN TEST- The client is in a standing position and the therapist is facing the client. The client will be asked to bring her arms into 90^0 of abduction and about 45^0 of horizontal adduction. From this position the client will be instructed to turn her arms as if she were emptying cans that are in her hands. Once the hands are in the position of having "emptied the cans" the therapist will apply a downward pressure on the arms (slight to moderate amount of pressure). If this reproduces the pain of which the client was complaining, it is likely that there is some degree of shoulder impingement.

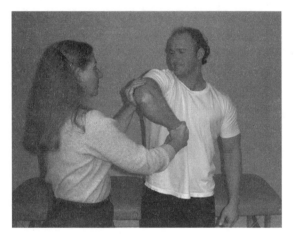

Figure 9-12c
The Hawkins-Kennedy Impingement sign examining for shoulder impingement.

HAWKINS-KENNEDY IMPINGEMENT SIGN- This is another valuable test to cross-reference for the presence of shoulder impingement. The client is in a standing position. The therapist will forward flex the client's shoulder to 90^0. From the position of forward flexion the therapist will then internally rotate the shoulder as far as it will go. This will bring the greater tuberosity of the humerus up under the coracoacromial arch and press on the soft-tissue structures under the arch. If there is impingement present, it is likely that this will reproduce the discomfort.

SUGGESTIONS FOR TREATMENT: Shoulder impingement can be well treated by massage approaches. It is important to establish, if possible, the tissues that are being impinged in order to determine the most effective treatment. For example, if the bursa is being impinged, the treatment might focus more on trying to reestablish the proper muscular balance around the shoulder joint so that the humerus is not pulled so far up into the glenoid fossa, thereby increasing the chance of impingement. If the impingement is primarily involving the supraspinatus tendon, deep transverse friction approaches may also be used in order to promote the proper development of functional scar tissue. Stretching and range of motion exercises will be helpful adjuncts. It will also be helpful to strengthen the muscles surrounding the shoulder joint so they can create optimum biomechanical balance.

biceps brachii tendon
(long head)

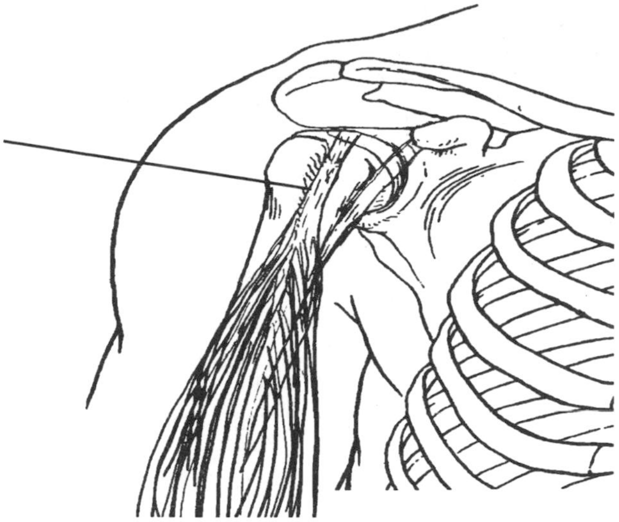

Figure 9-13a
*Anterior view of right shoulder
showing common site of bicipital
tendinitis between greater and
lesser tuberosities of humerus*

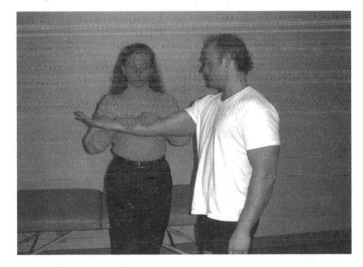

CHARACTERISTICS: The tendon of the long head of the biceps runs through a narrow groove in the upper humerus between the greater and lesser tuberosities. If this groove is relatively narrow or the individual engages in repeated motions of the shoulder which causes the tendon to rub against either the lessor or greater tuberosity, small micro tearing of the tendon will occur and tendinitis will develop.

ASSESSMENT: The client is likely to report pain in the shoulder which may be more localized toward the anterior portion of the shoulder. Pain is likely to increase with any activities that involve shoulder movements, especially if those movements involve shoulder flexion. Pain may also be elicited from movements of repeated elbow flexion or elbow flexion against a significant resistance such as lifting a heavy weight. There is also likely to be tenderness of the bicipital tendon in the anterior shoulder region. Bicipital tendinitis may become more evident in examination through the use of Speed's test.

Figure 9-13b
*Speed's test examining for
bicipital tendinitis.*

SPEED'S TEST- The client is in a standing position with the shoulder flexed to 90^0, the elbow fully extended and the palm supinated. The therapist will tell the client to hold the arm in this position while she exerts a downward force on the distal portion of the arm. If pain is felt in the anterior shoulder region, it is likely that there is some involvement with the bicipital tendon. A slight variation on this test which may also be used is to use an eccentric contraction of the biceps during the testing phase. This is done by instructing the client to slowly lower the arm from the beginning position while the therapist is exerting a downward pressure on the arm. The attempt to make this movement slow requires the biceps to work eccentrically.

SUGGESTIONS FOR TREATMENT: As with many other tendinitis conditions, the best method to address this condition involves decreasing tension in the offending muscle (biceps brachii). This is done effectively with massage. Stretching does not seem to be as effective for the biceps brachii because it is rarely limited in its elongation, and the full extension of the elbow prevents it from being able to be stretch much beyond its natural limit. Deep transverse friction can be applied to the bicipital tendon to enhance the development of a functionally mobile scar and the proper alignment of fibers during the repair phase. NOTE: Care should be taken when administering deep friction massage to the bicipital tendon. If the bicipital groove is shallow and the greater and lessor tuberosities are not very prominent it is possible to dislodge the tendon from the groove.

---

(76) CONDITION: PECTORALIS MINOR SYNDROME

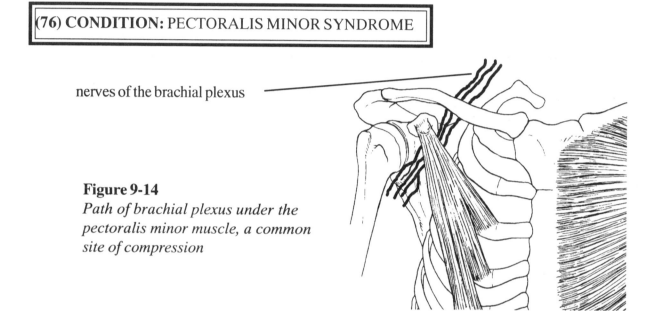

nerves of the brachial plexus

Figure 9-14
Path of brachial plexus under the pectoralis minor muscle, a common site of compression

CHARACTERISTICS: Symptoms of pectoralis minor syndrome are very similar to those of thoracic outlet syndrome because the mechanism of injury is very similar. Neurovascular structures are being compressed in the region of the upper brachial plexus. However, the location of the compression is slightly different. In pectoralis minor syndrome the compression is happening under the pectoralis minor muscle as it traps the neurovascular bundle against the upper rib cage. This is often caused by a tight pectoralis minor muscle in combination with other postural distortions such as the rounded shoulders described earlier in the chapter.

ASSESSMENT: The client will have symptoms such as pain, numbness, or paresthesia down the distribution of the arm. The pain or paresthesia will often be recognized along the distribution of the ulnar nerve which can be felt in the 4th and 5th fingers of the hand. The pain or paresthesia will often be elicited by bringing the arm into abduction past 90^0.

SUGGESTIONS FOR TREATMENT: It may be difficult to determine if the compression of the neurovascular bundle is happening at the thoracic outlet or under pectoralis minor. In that instance it is helpful to treat them both. This will also help achieve a better biomechanical balance. The pectoralis minor is deep underneath the pectoralis major and will not be responsive to superficial treatment. The best results with getting the pectoralis minor to release will come from deep longitudinal stripping techniques combined with stretching and postural reeducation.

(77) CONDITION: SUB-ACROMIAL BURSITIS

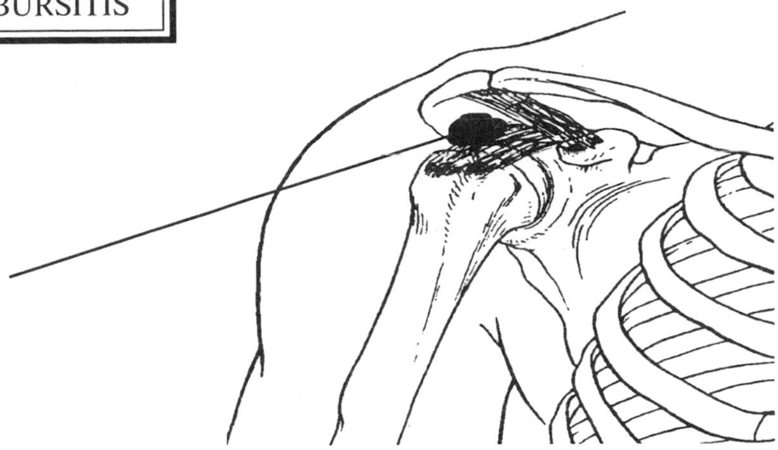

Figure 9-15
Anterior view of right shoulder showing location of sub-acromial bursa

CHARACTERISTICS: The sub-acromial bursa was mentioned along with shoulder impingement syndrome earlier. This is one of the more common locations of bursitis in the body. The sub-acromial bursa lies just below the acromion process in the shoulder. Repetitive motion, especially in full flexion or abduction, or direct trauma to the shoulder may cause the bursa to become inflamed. When the bursa is inflamed, motion at the shoulder will be painful.

ASSESSMENT: The client will present with factors in the history that point either to chronic overuse of the shoulder or perhaps a direct trauma on the point of the acromion process which may have caused the bursa to become inflamed. The client will most likely have pain with both passive and active motion in abduction at the shoulder and may exhibit a painful arc in abduction. A painful arc is represented by a certain range of motion that is painful. For example, a client may be able to abduct the arm to 45^0 with no pain. Pain begins at 45^0 of abduction and continues to 135^0 of abduction. After 135^0 there is no pain. The region between 45^0 and 135^0 is the painful arc. In many instances it may be hard to determine if the shoulder pain is coming from impingement of an irritated supraspinatus tendon or from the sub-acromial bursa.

SUGGESTIONS FOR TREATMENT: Bursitis is often treated with rest, and anti-inflammatory medication. The bursa will usually return to its normal state if the offending activity is stopped. Massage can play an important part in this although it is actually an indirect approach. Massage applications should be aimed at normalizing tension in the muscles of the shoulder girdle so the proper biomechanical function can be restored. Massage is not aimed at directly treating an inflamed bursa, but the indirect effect can be very helpful.

(78) CONDITION: GLENOHUMERAL DISLOCATION/SUBLUXATION

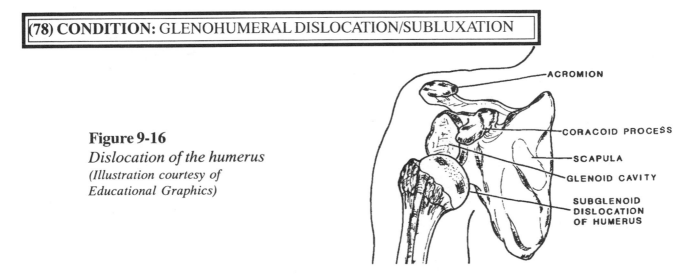

Figure 9-16
Dislocation of the humerus
(Illustration courtesy of Educational Graphics)

153   ANTERIOR VIEW

CHARACTERISTICS: The glenohumeral joint has a tremendous range of motion compared to many other joints in the body. The movements of the shoulder require that a greater range of motion be available. Although the great range of motion which is available at the glenohumeral joint is a distinct advantage in allowing freedom of movement, there is a potential drawback. By allowing greater range of motion, stability is sacrificed at the joint. There are not excessive ligamentous structures holding the joint firmly in place as in many other joints. In addition, the glenoid fossa is rather shallow and does not form a stable receptacle for the head of the humerus. It is mostly musculo-tendinous soft-tissues that keep the head of the humerus stable in the joint. A sudden force applied to the humerus may force the head of the humerus out of the glenoid fossa. An example of how this happens is when a person is falling. The natural inclination is to hold your arms out in front of you to break your fall. This may break your fall somewhat, but it also may force the head of the humerus out of the glenoid fossa. The most common dislocations or subluxations are in the anterior direction and result from the combined movements of abduction and external rotation of the shoulder.

A dislocation is where the head of the humerus is driven out of the glenohumeral joint and stays out of the joint. A subluxation is where the dislocation is only partial (the head of the humerus is not fully out of the joint) or the humerus may move out of the joint and quickly back in.

ASSESSMENT: If the humerus is dislocated it will usually be quite evident. There will be a history of a recent trauma to the shoulder joint. The client will not be able to move or use the arm without significant pain. The contour of the shoulder will appear significantly different than the other side as the humerus will usually be hanging lower. The susceptibility for dislocations can often be demonstrated during active and passive range of motion testing. If the client shows noticeable apprehension to particular motions of the shoulder and describes the sensation of feeling like the shoulder might "go out", this is an indication of instability being present.

SUGGESTIONS FOR TREATMENT: A shoulder dislocation or subluxation needs to be immediately put back into place (this is called a reduction). However, this needs to be done by someone who is trained to reduce dislocations because significant injury to the soft-tissues, such as arteries or nerves around the joint, can be done by incorrectly reducing the dislocation. A massage therapist will rarely be in the position to see a shoulder while it is still dislocated. However, knowledge about the potential for dislocation is very important while a treatment program is being designed. If a client has a history of shoulder dislocation, they may have recurrent shoulder instability. This instability will limit some of the things that you may want to do during your treatment or suggest for your client to do at home. For example, if a client has had recurrent anterior dislocations of the shoulder, it will not be a good idea to engage them in any mobilizations, massage procedures, or stretches that involve bringing the shoulder into a position of abduction and external rotation. Strengthening exercises will often be given for the muscles surrounding the joint to make up for the laxity of the joint.

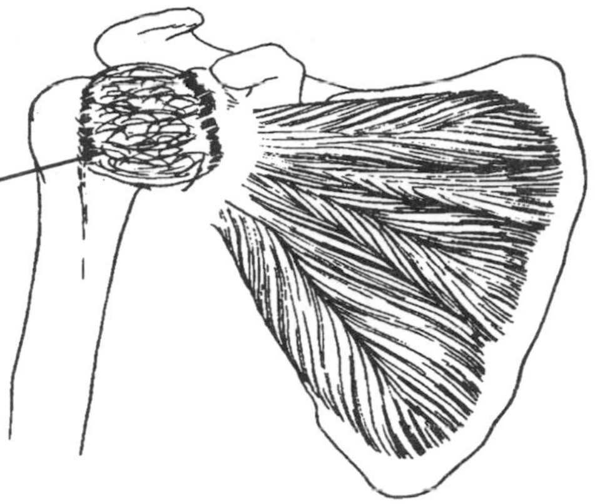

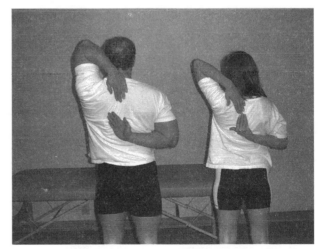

Figure 9-17a
*Anterior view of right
shoulder joint capsule*

FIBROUS ADHESIONS

CHARACTERISTICS: The glenohumeral joint is encased in a ligamentous joint capsule that helps provide some stability at the joint and house the synovial fluid that helps to lubricate the joint. The shoulder joint has a wide range of motion. It is often the joint capsule that is the primary factor in limiting the end range of motion for the shoulder in certain directions. Numerous factors including recent trauma, immobilization, or emotional stress can cause the joint capsule of the shoulder to become fibrous and adhere to adjacent tissues. When the capsule develops this fibrous adhesion to adjacent tissues (it may also adhere to itself between adjacent "folds"), it greatly limits mobility in the shoulder. The motions that are limited first in adhesive capsulitis are usually abduction and external rotation. This condition is often very long standing and slow to respond to treatment. Adhesive capsulitis occurs more often in women than in men.

ASSESSMENT: The client will often develop this condition over a long period of time. They will report limited range of motion and often display difficulty moving their shoulder into abduction and external rotation. When asked to abduct the arm, the client will often abduct the arm to a certain level and then continue attempting the abduction by raising the scapula or laterally flexing the torso. The available range of motion on each side can be examined by use of the Apley scratch test.

Figure 9-17b
The Apley scratch test examining for range of motion in each shoulder.

APLEY SCRATCH TEST- The client is in a standing position. One arm (the upper arm) will be in a position of abduction and external rotation. The other arm (the lower arm) will be in a position of adduction and internal rotation. It is a good idea to compare and contrast the available range of motion for both these actions between sides. It is not uncommon to see a greater range of motion on the non-dominant side.

SUGGESTIONS FOR TREATMENT: There are a number of approaches that can be used in treating

155

adhesive capsulitis. Massage is a very effective approach when used in conjunction with other range of motion, stretching, and strengthening activities. Massage is particularly effective because the change in tissue consistency that can be encouraged is slow and the results will tend to stay longer than an abrupt intervention. However, the practitioner and the client must often be patient, because the process can seem quite long. Some of the best results will be accomplished by using deep longitudinal stripping techniques on the anterior and posterior shoulder girdle muscles. Techniques that combine stripping with passive elongation of the affected tissues will enhance effects even more. In severe cases where the shoulder is not responsive to conservative treatment, a manipulation performed under anesthesia is often performed. This is done to try to forcibly elongate and "tear" the adhered fibers loose so the capsule can resume its free movement.

(80) CONDITION: MUSCLE STRAIN

CHARACTERISTICS: Acute overloading of musculotendinous structures in the shoulder will lead to muscle strains. Muscle strains in the shoulder tend to occur more often from high levels of eccentric loading. They don't tend to be as common here as in some other locations. However, when they do occur, the accessibility of the shoulder muscles makes them easier to treat.

ASSESSMENT: Knowledge of anatomy will be crucial in determining the presence of muscle strains. These conditions may have a number of symptoms depending on their severity. See the section in the beginning of the book on muscle strains for a more complete description of the differences between the various grades of strain. Determination of muscle pain or weakness may be based on the use of various manual resistive tests which isolate that muscle. Manual resistive tests for the six primary single plane movements of the shoulder were included at the beginning of this chapter.

SUGGESTIONS FOR TREATMENT: Any discussion of the treatment of muscle strains must be considered relative to the degree of the strain. For instance, the method of treatment for a grade 1 strain will be quite different from that of a severe grade 3 strain. In most instances muscle strains will be treated with rest from the offending activity, some type of anti-inflammatory treatment, stretching in the post-acute phase, and gradual strengthening as the injury repair progresses. Massage applications such as deep transverse friction are quite effective in helping to create a functional scar that is strong, yet pliable enough not to impair the proper use of the tissue. Massage is also very helpful during the rehabilitative phase to decrease muscle spasm which may have occurred immediately after the injury and is preventing the proper biomechanical balance from returning.

(81) CONDITION: NEUROMUSCULAR PAIN

CHARACTERISTICS: Any muscle in the body is capable of holding an increased level of neurological activity and maintaining a spasm. The spasm of that muscle will then lead to increased pain and disturbed biomechanical function. Muscle spasm can be perpetuated by various stimuli including chemicals like caffeine, certain medications, myofascial trigger points, or emotional stress. The pain may be relieved by rest, but simple activities of daily living will often cause the pain to resurface. The muscles of the shoulder girdle are quite susceptible to this type of stress, partly because of their mechanical and postural role.

ASSESSMENT: The muscles will frequently be painful in certain areas to palpation, may demonstrate a decreased range of motion, and may be somewhat painful on a resisted isometric contraction. They may contain painful myofascial trigger points which refer pain or other autonomic phenomena to remote areas. Familiarity with common trigger point pain referral patterns will aid in the determination of which shoulder muscles may be involved. Chronic overuse, postural or biomechanical imbalances which are evident through the history may be indicating factors. See the sections above for references on manual resistive tests and range of motion testing for selected muscles of the shoulder.

SUGGESTIONS FOR TREATMENT: These conditions respond very favorably to massage applications. Since muscular spasm is a primary component of these conditions, a technique like massage that is highly effective in addressing muscular spasm is very effective in reducing the complaint. If the condition arises from poor postural or biomechanical function, movement reeducation is very helpful, and in most cases necessary, as an adjunctive treatment.

Quick Reference for Conditions of the Shoulder

REGION OF PAIN	ONSET	POSSIBLE CAUSE	REF.
ANTERIOR SHOULDER	ACUTE	SHOULDER SEPARATION	72
LATERAL, ANTERIOR, OR POSTERIOR SHOULDER	ACUTE OR CHRONIC	ROTATOR CUFF TEAR	73
LATERAL SHOULDER (MAY FEEL LIKE IT IS IN THE JOINT)	CHRONIC	SHOULDER IMPINGEMENT SYNDROME	74
ANTERIOR SHOULDER	CHRONIC	BICIPITAL TENDINITIS	75
ARM, SHOULDER, HANDS	CHRONIC	PECTORALIS MINOR SYNDROME	76
LATERAL SHOULDER (MAY FEEL LIKE IT IS IN THE JOINT)	CHRONIC	SUB-ACROMIAL BURSITIS	77
SHOULDER JOINT	ACUTE	GLENOHUMERAL DISLOCATION/ SUBLUXATION	78
ENTIRE SHOULDER JOINT	CHRONIC	ADHESIVE CAPSULITIS	79
ANY MUSCLE	ACUTE OR CHRONIC	MUSCLE STRAIN	80
ANY MUSCLE	CHRONIC	NEUROMUSCULAR PAIN	81

CHAPTER 10

ELBOW, FOREARM, WRIST, & HAND CONDITIONS

Overview of Common Single Plane Movements of the Elbow

Active and passive ROM tests and manual resistive tests will require a knowledge of basic joint mechanics and functional anatomy for the regions surrounding the joint. The practitioner must know what constitutes normal, pain free motion in order to determine if there is a problem. The discussions of active ROM tests, passive ROM tests, and manual resistive tests will utilize the terms listed below. Familiarity with these terms and how they apply to the body will be essential in order to gain valid information from the assessment. All joint angle measurements which are included are measured from the neutral position, which is anatomical position. In order to properly understand and simplify joint mechanics, the movements at the joints have been broken down into single plane movements. That means movement in one of the three primary planes of motion - sagittal, frontal, or transverse. Although this greatly simplifies the analysis of movement it should be kept in mind that this classification rarely happens in actual human movement. Almost every movement we make will be a combination of movements in different planes. However, muscle or joint dysfunction can often be accurately pinpointed by comparing certain single plane movements. The primary muscles involved with each action are listed under the description of that action. Note that this may not include every muscle which is involved in that action, but only the primary ones.

Flexion- a movement at the elbow which brings the forearm toward the upper arm. Average range of motion for flexion is often dependent on the size of the arms, but will generally be about 145^0. The primary muscles used in flexion are:

> **Brachialis**
> **Biceps Brachii**
> **Brachioradialis**

Extension- the return to anatomical position from a position of flexion. In some individuals who have ligamentous laxity, a certain amount of movement may be gained that goes beyond anatomical position. This is hyperextension. Average range of motion in extension is considered 0^0 because that is complete extension. The primary muscles involved with extension are:

> **Triceps**
> **Anconeus**

NOTE: There are two additional movements, pronation and supination, which happen at the proximal radio-ulnar joint (at the elbow) in addition to the distal radioulnar joint (at the wrist). They will be covered in the section below on wrist movements.

Overview of Common Single Plane Movements of the Wrist

Flexion- a movement of the wrist which brings the palm toward the anterior surface of the forearm. Average range of motion for flexion is 85^0. The primary muscles used in flexion are:

Flexor Carpi Radialis
Flexor Carpi Ulnaris
Palmaris Longus

Extension- a movement that returns the wrist to anatomical position from any amount of flexion. If movement continues in the direction of extension past anatomical position the wrist is in hyperextension. Note that the average range of motion for wrist extension is all in hyperextension (i.e. measured from anatomical position). Average range of motion for wrist extension is 85^0. The primary muscles used in extension are:

Extensor Carpi Ulnaris
Extensor Carpi Radialis Brevis
Extensor Carpi Radialis Longus

Pronation- a movement of the wrist which is easiest to see if the elbow is held in 90^0 of flexion. From this position the palm of the hand faces directly downward. Average range of motion in pronation is 85^0. The primary muscles used in pronation are:

Pronator Quadratus
Pronator Teres

Supination- viewed from a position of 90^0 of elbow flexion, the palm is facing upward in the position that would be used to carry a tray. Average range of motion in supination is 90^0. The primary muscles used in supination are:

Supinator
Biceps Brachii

Radial Deviation/Abduction- the wrist moves in a frontal plane away from the midline of the body and the thumb moves toward the radius. Average range of motion in radial deviation is 15^0. The primary muscles used in radial deviation are:

Flexor carpi radialis
Palmaris Longus
Extensor Carpi Radialis Longus
Extensor Carpi Radialis Brevis

Ulnar Deviation/Adduction- is a movement of the wrist in which the hand (in anatomical position) moves in the frontal plane toward the midline of the body and the fifth finger moves toward the ulna. Average range of motion in ulnar deviation is 45^0. The primary muscles used in ulnar deviation are:

Flexor Carpi Ulnaris
Extensor Carpi Ulnaris

Active Range of Motion Tests

Active range of motion tests for the elbow will focus on flexion and extension. Active range of motion tests for the wrist will focus on the primary single plane movements of flexion, extension, pronation and supination. These movements will isolate all the major muscles acting on the wrist.

Passive Range of Motion Tests

Passive range of motion tests for the elbow will be relatively simple. The end-feel for flexion will be soft-tissue approximation, while the end-feel for extension will be bone-to-bone. At the wrist the mechanics of motion are more complex. There are a number of "floating" bones that are held together by a webbing of ligamentous structures. The motions that happen at the wrist joint are accomplished by small degrees of movement between these many different bones. The end-feel for flexion, extension, pronation, and supination will be most like tissue stretch. The end-feel for radial and ulnar deviation will be like an abrupt tissue stretch (ligamentous tissue stretching) almost similar to a bone-to-bone end-feel.

Manual Resistive Tests

The next section includes illustrations and descriptions of manual resistive tests for the two primary single plane movements of the elbow and the four primary movements of the wrist. Remember that each of these movements can be performed in either of the two ways described earlier to perform manual resistive tests.

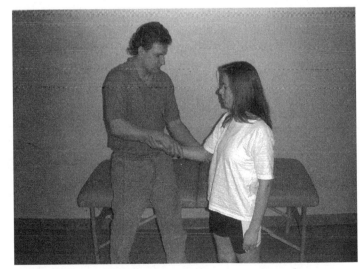

Figure 10-1
*Resisted flexion of
the elbow*

The client is in a standing or seated position with the elbow flexed to about 90^0. The therapist will place on hand on the elbow for stabilizing support and the other hand over the wrist. The client will be instructed to further flex the elbow while the therapist offers resistance.

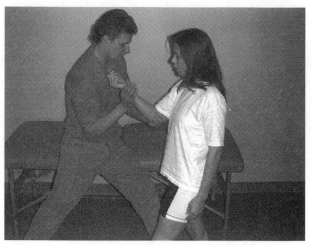

Figure 10-2
*Resisted extension
of the elbow*

The client is in a standing or seated position with the elbow flexed to about 120^0. The therapist has one hand on the elbow for stabilizing support and one hand underneath the wrist. The client will be instructed to hold the arm in that position as the therapist attempts to flex the elbow.

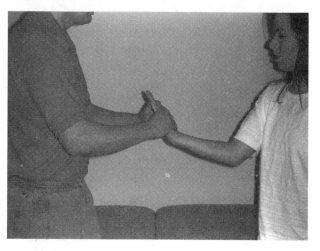

Figure 10-3
*Resisted flexion of
the wrist*

The client is in a standing or sitting position with the wrist supinated and slightly flexed and the elbow flexed to about 90^0. The therapist will grasp the client's hand with his fingers over the client's palm. The client will be instructed to flex the wrist further while the therapist offers resistance.

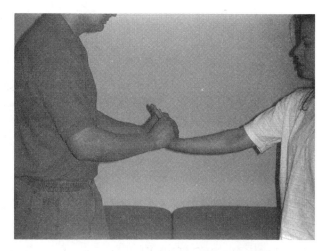

Figure 10-4
*Resisted extension
of the wrist*

The client is in a standing or sitting position with the wrist pronated and slightly hyperextended. The therapist will grasp the client's hand and place his fingers over the back side of the client's hand. The client will be instructed to extend the wrist further while the therapist offers resistance.

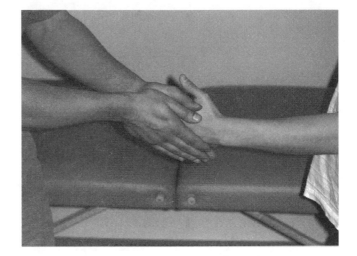

Figure 10-5
Resisted supination or pronation of the wrist. The starting position is the same for both.

The client is in a standing or sitting position with the wrist in a neutral position (thumb pointing up). The therapist will grasp the client's hand so that one hand is on the client's palm and one hand on the back of the client's hand. This position can be used for either pronation or supination. The therapist will instruct the client to hold the hand in this position while attempting to pronate (or supinate) the wrist. Remember that if the therapist is attempting to pronate the wrist, then the client is using the muscles of supination. Likewise, if the therapist is attempting to supinate the wrist, the client is using the muscles of pronation.

GUIDE TO CONDITIONS AND SPECIAL REGIONAL ORTHOPEDIC TESTS OF THE ELBOW, FOREARM, WRIST, AND HAND

Common Injury Conditions

(82) CONDITION: OLECRANON BURSITIS

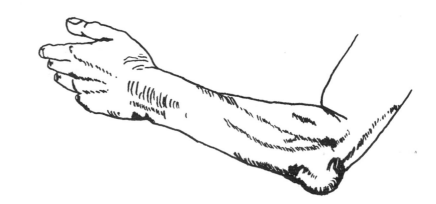

Figure 10-6
Olecranon bursitis. Swelling is very visible over the olecranon bursa.

CHARACTERISTICS: The olecranon bursa is a prominent bursa that sits between the skin and the olecranon process of the ulna. If it is subjected to a direct impact it is likely to become inflamed and produce olecranon bursitis. This may also occur if the individual irritates the bursa through chronic compression by constantly leaning on the elbows for example.

ASSESSMENT: This is one condition that is hard to miss. There is usually a visible area of swelling directly over the olecranon bursa that will be tender to touch. A history of direct trauma to the elbow or chronic compression will also be an indicator.

SUGGESTIONS FOR TREATMENT: The most effective treatments for olecranon bursitis will focus on reducing the inflammation. This may be done with ice or anti-inflammatory medications. In most instances, massage will not be an appropriate treatment for this condition. The bursa is quite superficial and additional compression of any kind may serve to irritate the bursa further. Massage may be beneficial in helping to keep tissue fluids moving out of the area, therefore helping to decrease any accumulation of edema.

---

(83) CONDITION: LATERAL HUMERAL EPICONDYLITIS (TENNIS ELBOW)

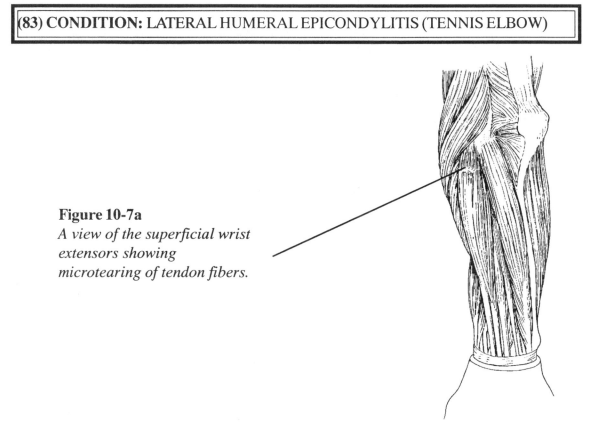

Figure 10-7a
A view of the superficial wrist extensors showing microtearing of tendon fibers.

CHARACTERISTICS: This condition involves trauma and microtearing of the tendon fibers of the common extensor tendons of the wrist where they attach to the lateral epicondyle of the humerus. This condition was first reported because of the frequency with which it affected tennis players. However, tennis players actually make up only a small portion of those individuals who have lateral humeral epicondylitis. The irritation and microtearing of the tendon fibers of the extensor group is mostly the result of <u>excessive eccentric loading</u> on the <u>extensors of the wrist</u>. The client will have pain, possibly some swelling, and limitation of movements that involve the wrist extensors. This condition frequently develops in occupational situations where people have to do repetitive flexion and extension motions of the wrist. *ECCENTRIC*

ASSESSMENT: The client will usually present with pain at the lateral region of the elbow that is associated with movement. They may feel pain on stretching the wrist extensor group (in full flexion of the wrist) and the region may be tender to palpation. There will usually be something in the history that indicates a repetitive motion that has overused the wrist extensors. The presence of lateral humeral epicondylitis can be further clarified by use of the tennis elbow test.

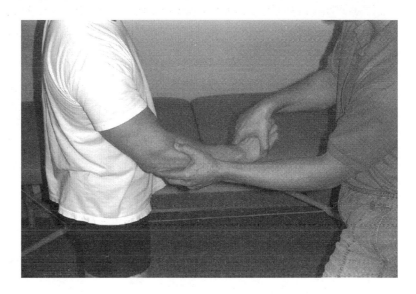

Figure 10-7b
Tennis elbow test examining for lateral humeral epicondylitis

TENNIS ELBOW TEST- The client is in a standing or sitting position. The therapist has one hand placed on the lateral elbow region. The thumb of that hand is directly over the common tendons of the wrist extensor muscles. Notice that the thumb will be distal to the lateral epicondyle of the humerus. The client will hold the wrist in about 45⁰ of extension (hyperextension). The therapist will instruct the client to hold the wrist in that position while he (the therapist) tries to bring the wrist into flexion. At the same time that he is trying to bring the client's wrist into flexion, he will be pressing on the common extensor tendons of the wrist with the thumb of his other hand. If this causes pain and discomfort at the lateral elbow region under the therapist's thumb, it is likely that there is some level of epicondylitis present. Notice that you may produce discomfort in someone who is completely non-symptomatic with this test. That does not mean that they have the condition, but the condition may be with them at a sub-clinical level which gives them a greater predisposition to developing a full-blown case of it at a later date.

SUGGESTIONS FOR TREATMENT: Lateral humeral epicondylitis is most often treated with rest from the offending activity and anti-inflammatory measures. The anti-inflammatory measures may include medications, ice applications, or other modalities. Bracing of the affected area is often used to enhance the mechanical support of the extensor tendons. The use of bracing will also enhance proprioception. By enhancing proprioception (the client's awareness of the area) they can pay more attention to making sure they use proper mechanics in motions that may irritate the area. Massage is quite effective in treating this condition. A combination of different techniques will yield good results. Deep transverse friction will be used to help properly align any scar tissue that is developing. Stripping massage techniques with active and passive movements for the wrist flexors and extensors will help to restore the proper biomechanical balance to the area, and decrease the mechanical loading on the tendons that causes the microtearing to occur.

— FREEZE STYROFOAM CUPS WITH WATER APPLY DIRECTLY TO AREA
— ALSO USE TRIGGER POINTS WHERE APPLICABLE

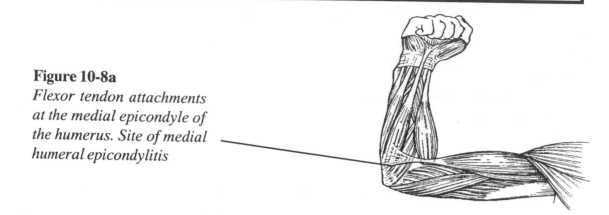

Figure 10-8a
Flexor tendon attachments at the medial epicondyle of the humerus. Site of medial humeral epicondylitis

CHARACTERISTICS: The characteristics for this condition are very similar to lateral epicondylitis except for the location of the pain and the muscle group which is responsible for the problem. In this condition the location of the pain is at the medial epicondyle of the humerus and the muscle group which causes the problem is the wrist flexors. This condition is not as common as lateral epicondylitis, but the way in which the injury develops is very similar. This condition is mostly a result of chronic eccentric loading on the wrist flexor group which causes irritation and microtearing of the tendon fibers. The condition is called golfer's elbow because of the frequency with which it is seen in people who play golf.

ASSESSMENT: The client will usually have something in their history that indicates chronic overloading of the wrist flexor group. Pain will be felt around the medial region of the elbow, especially with stretching of the wrist flexor group (full hyperextension of the wrist). The area may also be tender to palpation. The presence of medial humeral epicondylitis can be further clarified by use of the golfer's elbow test.

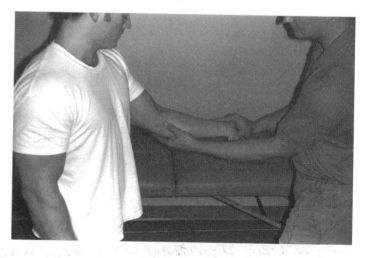

Figure 10-8b
Golfer's elbow test examining for medial humeral epicondylitis

GOLFER'S ELBOW TEST- The client is standing or sitting. The therapist has one hand on the elbow region with the thumb of that hand placed directly over the flexor tendons of the wrist. The other hand is over the client's palm which is in about 20^0 to 30^0 of (hyper) extension. The client will be instructed to hold the palm in that position while the therapist attempts to extend the wrist further. While attempting to extend the wrist, the therapist will also press on the flexor tendons just distal to the medial epicondyle of the humerus. If this elicits pain at the region of the medial epicondyle under the therapist's thumb, it is likely that there is a degree of medial epicondylitis present.

SUGGESTIONS FOR TREATMENT: See the suggestions for treatment listed under lateral epicondylitis. The methods of treatment will be very similar. The major difference is that any treatment methods that are specifically aimed at the lateral extensor tendons such as deep transverse friction will be aimed at the medial flexor tendons in this condition.

---

(85) CONDITION: CARPAL TUNNEL SYNDROME

Figure 10-9a
Anterior view of the palm showing the flexor retinaculum. The flexor tendons and the median nerve lie just beneath it.

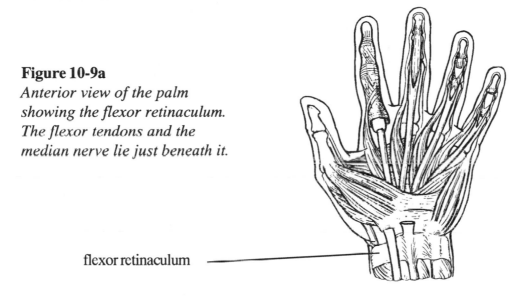

flexor retinaculum

CHARACTERISTICS: The presence of carpal tunnel syndrome is becoming more and more prevalent. This increase is often attributed to the dramatic increase in occupations involving repetitive motions, especially flexion motions of the fingers and hands. This is a nerve compression syndrome which is created by compression of the median nerve in the anterior region of the wrist. A tunnel is formed in the wrist by the carpal bones which make up the "roof" of the tunnel and a soft-tissue band called the flexor retinaculum (also called the transverse carpal ligament), which makes up the "floor" of the tunnel. The tunnel is shared by the median nerve and the tendons of hand and wrist flexors. Due to overuse, the tendons of the flexor muscles will swell within this tunnel. When they swell, they press on the median nerve causing pain, numbness, and lack of motor function.

ASSESSMENT: The client will most often present with some factors in the history that indicate repetitive use of the finger and hand flexor muscle group. If there are no factors present which indicate overuse of this muscle group, the condition may also be caused by the tendons getting irritated from remaining in a flexed position for long periods. The client will complain of pain in the anterior wrist and palmar surface of the hand. The pain will mostly be localized to the 1st, 2nd, & 3rd fingers of the hand. The pain may also be accompanied by numbness, paresthesia, or motor weakness (this will show up as a weakness or lack of grip strength). The presence of carpal tunnel syndrome can be further clarified by use of two special orthopedic tests: the Phalen's test and Tinel's sign.

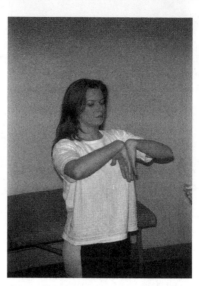

Figure 10-9b
Phalen's test examining for carpal tunnel syndrome

PHALEN'S TEST - The client places both wrists together with the dorsal surface of the hands resting against each other. The wrists should be held in a position of maximum flexion. The client will then be instructed to press the wrists together and hold them in that position for about 60 seconds. If this produces pain, numbness, or paresthesia in the palm, 2nd, 3rd, or 4th fingers, this may indicate the presence of carpal tunnel syndrome.

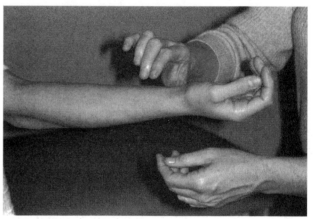

Figure 10-9c
Tinel's sign examining for carpal tunnel syndrome

TINEL'S SIGN - The therapist will supinate the client's hand and lightly tap on the anterior surface of the wrist. If this produces pain, numbness, or paresthesia along the distribution of the median nerve, it is indicative of carpal tunnel syndrome.

SUGGESTIONS FOR TREATMENT: Carpal tunnel syndrome is treated in a number of different ways. The most effective treatments will employ rest from the offending activity and some method of decreasing the inflammation of the flexor tendons. This may be accomplished through ice applications or the use of anti-inflammatory medication. Massage applications can be successful in treating the condition. Massage should focus on decreasing any accumulated tension in the flexor muscles of the wrist. Deep stripping techniques will often be effective in accomplishing this. Massage should also be applied further up the kinetic chain (arms, shoulder, or neck). It may not seem apparent at first, but tightness in these other areas can be a major contributing factor to a condition such as carpal tunnel syndrome.

If conservative measures are not successful in treating carpal tunnel syndrome, surgery is used to release compression on the median nerve. This is done by cutting the flexor retinaculum in order to make more room in the tunnel. However, the problems associated with overuse must eventually be addressed or the condition is likely to resurface at a later time.

(86) CONDITION: DeQUERVAIN'S TENOSYNOVITIS

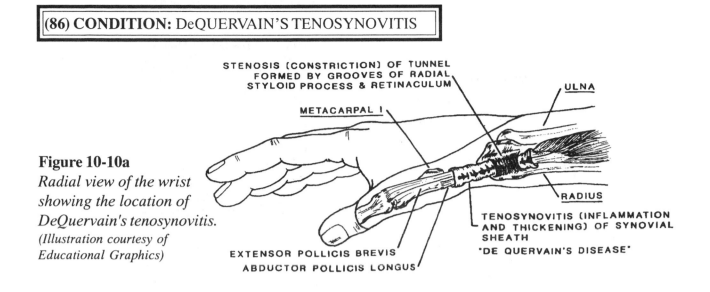

STENOSIS (CONSTRICTION) OF TUNNEL
FORMED BY GROOVES OF RADIAL
STYLOID PROCESS & RETINACULUM

ULNA

METACARPAL I

Figure 10-10a
*Radial view of the wrist
showing the location of
DeQuervain's tenosynovitis.*
(Illustration courtesy of
Educational Graphics)

RADIUS

TENOSYNOVITIS (INFLAMMATION
AND THICKENING) OF SYNOVIAL
SHEATH
'DE QUERVAIN'S DISEASE'

EXTENSOR POLLICIS BREVIS
ABDUCTOR POLLICIS LONGUS

RADIAL VIEW

CHARACTERISTICS: This condition involves overuse of the hand and wrist. There are two tendons located near the styloid process of the radius in an area known as the anatomical snuff box. They are the abductor pollicis longus and the extensor pollicis brevis. These tendons have a sheath surrounding them in order to protect them from excessive friction during movements of the wrist. If they are exposed to chronic overuse, they are likely to develop adhesion and irritation between the tendons and their sheaths. This is tenosynovitis.

ASSESSMENT: The client will have a history of some type of overuse that is affecting the hand. There will usually be pain and tenderness reported near the styloid process of the radius. This area may be tender to palpation and it is likely that movements of the wrist involving ulnar deviation will cause pain in the same region. Further clarification about the presence of DeQuervain's tenosynovitis can be gained by using the Finklestein test.

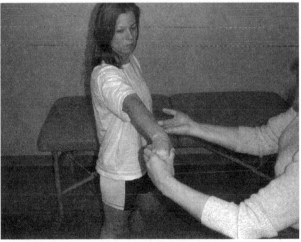

Figure 10-10b
*Finklestein test examining for
DeQuervain's tenosynovitis*

FINKLESTEIN TEST- The client is instructed to make a fist with the thumb tucked underneath the fingers. The client's wrist will then be moved (by either the client or the therapist) into a position of ulnar deviation. If this causes pain in the region of the anatomical snuff box at the radial styloid, it is likely that DeQuervain's tenosynovitis might be involved.

169

SUGGESTIONS FOR TREATMENT: This condition is treated similar to many other tenosynovitis conditions. Rest from or modification of the offending activity will be important. Anti-inflammatory treatments will be directed at decreasing any buildup of edema in the area. Deep friction massage specifically addressed to the abductor pollicis longus and the extensor pollicis brevis will be encouraged. Massage applications to the rest of the muscles acting on the wrist will also be beneficial in maintaining proper biomechanical balance.

(87) CONDITION: MUSCLE STRAIN

CHARACTERISTICS: Acute overloading of musculotendinous structures will lead to muscle strains. Muscle strains in the elbow, forearm, wrist, and hand tend to occur more often from high levels of eccentric loading. They don't tend to be as common here as in some other locations. The majority of muscle strains that will occur in these regions will manifest as small tears at the musculotendinous junction. Muscles involved in larger forces such as the biceps brachii are an exception.

ASSESSMENT: Knowledge of anatomy will be crucial in determining the presence of muscle strains. These conditions may have a number of symptoms depending on their severity. See the section in the beginning of the book on muscle strains for a more complete description of the differences between the various grades of strain. Determination of muscle pain or weakness may be based on the use of various manual resistive tests which isolate that muscle. Manual resistive tests for the primary single plane movements of the elbow and wrist were included at the beginning of this chapter.

SUGGESTIONS FOR TREATMENT: Any discussion of the treatment of muscle strains must be considered relative to the degree of the strain. For instance, the method of treatment for a grade 1 strain will be different from that of a severe grade 3 strain. In most instances muscle strains will be treated with rest from the offending activity, some type of anti-inflammatory treatment, stretching in the post-acute phase, and gradual strengthening as the injury repair progresses. Massage applications such as deep transverse friction are quite effective in helping to create a functional scar that is strong, yet pliable enough not to impair the proper use of the tissue. Massage is also very helpful during the rehabilitative phase to decrease muscle spasm which may have occurred immediately after the injury and is preventing the proper biomechanical balance from returning.

(88) CONDITION: NEUROMUSCULAR PAIN

CHARACTERISTICS: Any muscle in the body is capable of holding an increased level of neurological activity and maintaining a spasm. The spasm of that muscle will then lead to increased pain and disturbed biomechanical function. Muscle spasm can be perpetuated by various stimuli including chemicals like caffeine, certain medications, myofascial trigger points, or emotional stress. The pain may be relieved by rest, but simple activities of daily living will often cause the pain to resurface. The muscles of the shoulder girdle are quite susceptible to this type of stress, partly because of their mechanical and postural role.

ASSESSMENT: The muscles will frequently be painful in certain areas to palpation, may demonstrate a decreased range of motion, and may be somewhat painful on a resisted isometric contraction. They may contain painful myofascial trigger points which refer pain or other autonomic phenomena to remote areas. Familiarity with common trigger point pain referral patterns will aid in the determination of which muscles may be involved. Chronic overuse, postural, or biomechanical imbalances which are evident through the history may be indicating factors. See the sections above for references on manual resistive tests and range of motion testing for selected muscles of this region.

SUGGESTIONS FOR TREATMENT: These conditions respond very favorably to massage applications. Since muscular spasm is a primary component of these conditions, a technique like massage that is highly effective in addressing muscular spasm is very effective in reducing the complaint. If the condition arises from poor postural or biomechanical function, movement reeducation is very helpful, and in most cases necessary, as an adjunctive treatment.

— WEEN OFF CAFFIENE (DEHYDRATION) (CHEM STIMULATES)
— DRINK LOTS OF WATER

Quick Reference for Conditions of the Elbow, Forearm, Wrist, and Hand

REGION OF PAIN	ONSET	POSSIBLE CAUSE	REF.
POSTERIOR ELBOW	ACUTE OR CHRONIC	OLECRANON BURSITIS	82
LATERAL ELBOW	CHRONIC	LATERAL HUMERAL EPICONDYLITIS	83
MEDIAL ELBOW	CHRONIC	MEDIAL HUMERAL EPICONDYLITIS	84
WRIST, HAND, FINGERS	CHRONIC	CARPAL TUNNEL SYNDROME	85
RADIAL SIDE OF WRIST	CHRONIC	DeQUERVAIN'S TENOSYNOVITIS	86
ANY MUSCLE	ACUTE OR CHRONIC	MUSCLE STRAIN	87
ANY MUSCLE	CHRONIC	NEUROMUSCULAR PAIN	88

References and Suggested Reading

American Academy of Orthopaedic Surgeons: *Athletic Training and Sports Medicine, 2nd edition*, AAOS, 1991, ISBN 0-89203-044-5.

Booher, James & Thibodeau, Gary: *Athletic Injury Assessment, 2nd edition,* Times Mirror/ Mosby, 1989, ISBN 0-8016-2561-0.

Cailliet, Rene: *Low Back Pain Syndrome*, F.A. Davis, 1988, ISBN 0-8036-1606-6.

Cailliet, Rene: *Soft-Tissue Pain and Disability*, F. A. Davis, 1988, ISBN 0-8036-1631-7.

Chaitow, Leon: *Palpatory Literacy*, Thorsons, 1991, ISBN 0-7225-2198-7.

Chaitow, Leon: *Soft-Tissue Manipulation*, Healing Arts Press, 1980, ISBN 0-89281-276-1.

Clemente, Carmine: *Anatomy, 3rd edition*, Urban & Schwarzenberg, 1981, ISBN - 0-8067-0322-9.

Cyriax, J. & Cyriax, P.: *Illustrated Manual of Orthopaedic Medicine*, Butterworths, 1983, ISBN 0-407-00262-6.

Cyriax, James: *Textbook of Orthopaedic Medicine, 8th edition*, Balliere Tindall, 1982, ISBN 0-7020-0935-0.

Enoka, Roger: *Neuromechanical Basis of Kinesiology*, Human Kinetics, 1988, ISBN 0-87322-179-6.

Hartley, Anne: *Practical Joint Assessment*, Mosby Year Book, 1991, ISBN 0-8016-2050-3.

Hoppenfeld, Stanley: *Physical Examination of the Spine and Extremities*, Appleton & Lange, 1976, ISBN 0-8385-7853-5.

Kapandji, I.A.: *The Physiology of the Joints, Vols. 1,2, & 3*, Churchill Livingstone, 1982 (vol. 1), 1987 (vol. 2), 1974 (vol. 3), ISBN 0-443-02504-5 (vol. 1), 0-443-03618-7 (vol. 2), 0-443-01209-1 (vol. 3).

Kendall, Florence, McCreary, Elizabeth, & Provance, Patricia: *Muscles: Testing and Function*, Williams & Wilkins, 1993, ISBN 0-683-04576-8.

Kessler, Randolph & Hertling, Darlene: *Management of Common Musculoskeletal Disorders*, Harper & Row, 1983, ISBN 0-06-141429-8.

Luttgens, Kathryn & Wells, Katherine: *Kinesiology, 7th edition*, Saunders College Publishing, 1982, ISBN 0-03-058358-6.

Magee, David: ***Orthopedic Physical Assessment, 2nd edition***, W.B. Saunders, 1992, ISBN 0-7216-4344-2.

Netter, Frank: ***Atlas of Human Anatomy***, Ciba-Geigy, 1989, ISBN 0-914168-18-5.

Nordin, Margareta & Frankel, Victor: ***Basic Biomechanics of the Musculoskeletal System, 2nd edition***, Lea & Febiger, 1989, ISBN 0-8121-1227-X.

Norkin, Cynthia, & Levangie, Pamela: ***Joint Structure and Function***, F.A. Davis, 1983, ISBN 0-8036-6576-8.

Prentice, William: ***Rehabilitation Techniques in Sports Medicine***, Times Mirror/Mosby, 1990, ISBN 0-8016-6147-1.

Prudden, Bonnie: ***Pain Erasure***, Ballantine Books, 1980, ISBN 0-345-33102-8.

Roy, Steven & Irvin, Richard: ***Sports Medicine, Prevention, Evaluation, Management, and Rehabilitation***, Prentice Hall, 1983, ISBN 0-13-837807-X.

Sieg, Kay, & Adams, Sandra: ***Illustrated Essentials of Musculoskeletal Anatomy, 2nd edition***, Megabooks, 1985, ISBN 0-935157-00X.

Stone, Robert J. & Stone, Judith A.: ***Atlas of the Skeletal Muscles***, William C. Brown, 1990, ISBN 0-697-10618-7.

Torg, Joseph S. & Shephard, Roy J.: ***Current Therapy in Sports Medicine***, Mosby, 1995, ISBN 1-55664-384-5.

Travell, Janet & Simons, David: ***Myofascial Pain & Dysfunction, The Trigger Point Manual, Volumes 1 & 2***, Williams & Wilkins, 1983 (vol.1), 1992 (vol. 2), ISBN 0-683-08366-X (vol. 1), ISBN 0-683-08367-8 (vol. 2).

Wadsworth, Carolyn T.: ***Manual Examination and Treatment of the Spine and Extremities***. Williams & Wilkins, 1988, ISBN 0-683-08600-6.

Index

T

Tailor's bunion 50
Tarsal tunnel syndrome 53
Tendinitis *16*
Tendon *11, 15*
   avulsion *17*
Tennis elbow 164
Tennis elbow test 165
Tenosynovitis *16*
Tensile stress *15, 16, 18*
Tension *5*
Tensor Fasciae Latae 94
Teres Major 139, 140, 141
Teres Minor 139, 140, 141
Test
   Achilles tendon pinch test 55
   Active range of motion 27
   Adson maneuver 132
   Ankle drawer sign 58
   Apley compression test 81
   Apley distraction test 81
   Apley scratch test 155
   Cervical compression 135
   Cervical traction 135
   Clarke's sign 84
   Cross over test 147
   Empty can test 150
   FABER test102
   Finklestein test 169
   Gapping test 102
   Hawkins-Kennedy impingement sign 150
   Lachman test 76
   Manual resistive test *33*
   Noble compression test 89
   Ober test 88
   Passive range of motion *30*
   Patellofemoral compression test 84
   Piriformis test 104
   Posterior drawer test 77
   Special regional orthopedic tests *35*
   Speed's test 151
   Straight leg raise test 117
   Tennis elbow test 165
   Thomas test 98
   Thompson test 57
   Valgus stress test 78
   Varus stress test 80
Tests
   active range of motion *26*
   manual resistive tests *26*
   passive range of motion *26*
   special regional orthopedic *27*
Third degree *14*
Thomas test 98
Thompson test 57
Thoracic outlet syndrome 131

Tibial nerve 53
Tibialis Anterior 40, 41
Tibialis Posterior 40, 41
TINEL'S SIGN 168
Tissue
   contractile *11*
   inert *11*
   mechanical disruption *4*
   neurological dysfunction *7*
Torsion *5*
Torticollis 133
Transverse Abdominus 110
Transverse arch 39
Transversospinalis 110
Trapezius 126
Triceps 139, 159
Triceps (long head) 139
triceps surae *16*
Trochanteric bursitis 100

U

Ulnar deviation 161

V

Valgus stress test 78
Varus stress test 80
Vastus Intermedius 70
Vastus Lateralis 70
Vastus Medialis 70
VMO 69, 82

W

Whiplash 132

X

X-RAY *36*